Myths in

Medicine

Volume 1

Daniel G. Ostermayer, MD
McGovern Medical School
University of Texas Health Sciences Center at Houston
Department of Emergency Medicine

Ryan Pedigo, MD
Harbor UCLA Medical Center
Department of Emergency Medicine

Benjamin L. Cooper, MD
University of Texas Health Sciences Center at Houston
McGovern Medical School
Department of Emergency Medicine

ASSOCIATE EDITOR

Daniel P. Runde MD, MME
University of Iowa Hospitals and Clinics
Carver College of Medicine
Department of Emergency Medicine

ASSISTANT EDITOR

Manpreet Singh, MD
Harbor UCLA Medical Center
Department of Emergency Medicine

CHAPTER AUTHORS

Omid Adibnazari, MD
Harbor UCLA Medical Center
Department of Emergency Medicine

Tom Fadial, MD
McGovern Medical School
University of Texas Health Sciences Center at Houston
Department of Emergency Medicine

Alexander Garrett, MD
Harbor UCLA Medical Center
Department of Emergency Medicine

Jonathan Giordano, DO
McGovern Medical School
University of Texas Health Sciences Center at Houston
Department of Emergency Medicine

Alexander S. Grohmann, MD
Harbor UCLA Medical Center
Department of Emergency Medicine

Joshua Gross, MD
Medical College of Wisconsin
Department of Emergency Medicine

Evan Laveman, MD
Harbor UCLA Medical Center
Department of Emergency Medicine

Jennifer Lee, MD
Harbor UCLA Medical Center
Department of Emergency Medicine

Jason A. Lesnick, MD
McGovern Medical School
University of Texas Health Sciences Center at Houston
Department of Emergency Medicine

Nikhil R. Patel, MD
McGovern Medical School
University of Texas Health Sciences Center at Houston
Department of Emergency Medicine

Huy A. Phan, MD
McGovern Medical School
University of Texas Health Sciences Center at Houston
Department of Emergency Medicine

Kian Preston-Suni, MD MPH
Harbor UCLA Medical Center
Department of Emergency Medicine

Kerollos A. Shaker, MD
McGovern Medical School
University of Texas Health Sciences Center at Houston
Department of Emergency Medicine

Jackie Shibata, MD
Harbor UCLA Medical Center
Department of Emergency Medicine

Christopher T. Stephens, MD
McGovern Medical School
University of Texas Health Sciences Center at Houston
Department of Anesthesiology

Irma T. Ugalde, MD
McGovern Medical School
University of Texas Health Sciences Center at Houston
Department of Emergency Medicine

John C. Waller-Delarosa, MD
McGovern Medical School
University of Texas Health Sciences Center at Houston
Department of Emergency Medicine

James H. Williams, MD
Harbor UCLA Medical Center
Department of Emergency Medicine

Richard B. Witkov, MD
McGovern Medical School
University of Texas Health Sciences Center at Houston
Department of Emergency Medicine

Myths in Emergency Medicine examines the origin, facts, and misconceptions of many common bedside teachings. These are some of the oldest and most pervasive medical myths. With each topic we discuss the best available evidence to guide clinical care, and acknowledge the areas of continued uncertainty. Ironically, disproving a myth may actually create a new myth, but these common tales are filled with many falsehoods. By taking a deep dive into these common myths we hope you will both gain an appreciation for medical history and improve your clinical practice and skepticism. Please perform your own research prior to changing personal clinical practice.

Null Publishing
Group

Null Publishing Group, an academic publisher, provides tools, resources, and expertise to authors publishing educational texts. Authors retain ownership and control, and choose the desired copyright of their published works, while gaining the flexibility and power of digital publishing.

A penicillin allergy contraindicates administration of cephalosporins

Daniel G. Ostermayer

The Origin

During the 1980s, penicillin G and cephalosporins were produced with the same fungi, and trace amounts of penicillin contaminated cephalosporin preparations.[1] This increased the likelihood of patients receiving a penicillin-contaminated cephalosporin and potentially experiencing an allergic reaction. The possibility of contamination caused the allergy cross-reactivity of all cephalosporins to be reported at 10% of those with a penicillin allergy. In addition, first- and second-generation cephalosporins share a similar side chain, which may increase the likelihood of allergic cross-reactivity.[2] An alert has since been programed into warning messages within electronic medical records to alert providers when ordering a cephalosporin for any patient with a penicillin allergy.

The Facts

The cross-reactivity between cephalosporins and penicillins is significantly lower than 10%. Observational studies found cross-reactivity rates of between 0.17% and 0.7% while a prospective study reported rates as high as 6%.[3,4] Although cross-reactivity between penicillins and cephalosporins is most likely associated with structurally similar side chains rather than the beta-lactam ring itself, the incidence was exaggerated due to the manufacturing contamination that occurred in the past. For example, cefadroxil, a first generation cephalosporin shares the same side-chain as amoxicillin and has the greatest cross-reactivity rate (27%).[5] The later the generation of cephalosporin, the less side chain similarity to penicillin and synthetic penicillins, and the lower the likelihood of cross-reactivity. A meta-analysis calculated a rate of 1-10% for first-generation cephalosporins and negligible rates with second- and third-generation cephalosporins.[6]

Despite the widespread perception of high penicillin allergy prevalence, many can have their self-reported allergy removed after more careful clinical review due to lack of severe allergic symptoms.[7,8] Pairing the rare cephalosporin cross-reactivity with the greatly exaggerated rate of penicillin allergies make administration of cephalosporins, especially second-generation or later, most likely safe. Alternative antibiotics should still be used if the patient reports anaphylaxis, in order to err on the side of extreme caution.

The Bottom Line

- Most patient overestimate their penicillin allergy and verification of the allergic symptoms is important for accurate allergy profiling.
- Penicillin and cephalosporins cross-reactivities are far less than the originally reported 10% and negligible (probably less than 2%) for second-generation cephalosporins and later.

- Historic penicillin production problems resulted in contamination of cephalosporins.
- First generation cephalosporins share a similar side chain with penicillin that may increase the risk of cross-reactivity.

Use sterile gloves for all laceration repairs

Joshua Gross, Daniel G. Ostermayer

The Origin

With nearly 12 million patients requiring wound care annually, laceration repairs are the second most common procedure performed in the emergency department.[9] Traditional and historical practices have long recommended sterile gloves for uncomplicated laceration exploration and repair, with the underlying motivation being the minimization of secondary wound infection.[10] Theoretically, maximizing sterility of all equipment including gloves could decrease the risk of inoculating a wound during laceration repair.

The Facts

In the 1980s, several studies challenged the notion that sterile gloves decrease the likelihood of wound infection during laceration repair. The data suggested that nonsterile gloves did not increase the infection rate when compared to sterile gloves.[11,12]

Infection rates range from 3.5% to 7% of wounds and lacerations treated in emergency departments.[13,14] In 2004, a landmark randomized controlled trial evaluated the effect of clean, nonsterile gloves on laceration infection rates. The multicenter trial compared the use of individually packaged sterile gloves to clean nonsterile gloves for uncomplicated laceration repair in the emergency department. For the 816 randomized patients, the study did not find a statistically significant difference in the incidence of wound infection between the two groups. The infection rate for nonsterile clean gloves was 4.4% versus 6.1% for sterile gloves.[15] Lacerations classified as uncomplicated included those without signs of infection, neurovascular compromise, tendon injury, foreign bodies, open fractures, bites, or delayed presentation (>12 hours), and those in patients without diabetes or immunocompromised state. Although certainly suggestive of safe practice with nonsterile gloves for laceration repairs, the broad exclusion criteria make extrapolation to all ED patients impossible.

An additional study even analyzed the degree of bacterial colonization in unused sterile versus nonsterile clean gloves. In an outpatient clinic minor procedure room, unused sterile gloves had a lower bacterial load than unused nonsterile clean gloves, but neither contained the bacterial concentration ($>10^5$ organisms/mL)[16] necessary to cause a subsequent wound infection through direct innoculation.[17]

For complicated wounds, or complex repairs where a closely fitted glove may aid repair, sterile gloves may be preferred.

The Bottom Line

- Uncomplicated wounds have 3.5%–7% risk of infection after emergency department laceration repair.
- Repairing these uncomplicated lacerations with standard nonsterile gloves does not increase the infectious risk compared to sterile surgical gloves.

- For complicated wounds, or complex repairs where a closely fitted glove may aid repair, sterile gloves may be preferred.

Arterial blood gas is superior to a venous blood gas

Benjamin L. Cooper, Jason A. Lesnick

The Origin

Arterial blood leaves the left ventricle after pulmonary oxygenation and has minimal to no peripheral tissue oxygen extraction. Traditionally, clinicians are taught that an arterial blood gas (ABG) sample serves as the reference standard for pH, oxygen, carbon dioxide, and lactate content. The relationship between venous and arterial blood gas sampling has been studied for more than half a century.[18] There is little debate on the agreement of arterial and venous blood gas samples under normal physiologic conditions, but myths and controversy emerged regarding the relationship between arterial and venous measurements under conditions of physiologic stress and critical illness.

In the mid to late 1980s, *The New England Journal of Medicine* published two studies that demonstrated large differences between central venous and arterial blood gas measurements of patients with circulatory failure. They concluded that both arterial and central venous blood gases were important but served different roles. While the arterial blood gas provided information regarding pulmonary gas exchange, the venous blood gas more accurately reflected the tissue milieu—more acidic and hypercarbic.[19,20] The discrepancies between arterial and venous blood gas samples in critically ill patients contributed to a misconception that arterial blood gases were always required for accurate clinical decision making.

The Facts

While arterial samples have some diagnostic utility, they are painful for the patient, increase risks of bleeding, infection, nerve injury, digital ischemia, and injury to staff, and can require significantly more time.[21] Although venous sampling does not provide the most accurate reflection of pulmonary gas exchange, a venous partial pressure of carbon dioxide (pCO_2) of less than or equal to 45 mmHg is 100% sensitive for ruling out arterial hypercarbia (defined as arterial $pCO_2 > 45$ mmHg).[22]

Also, venous sampling does not provide the most accurate measurement of a patient's ability to oxygenate. A reliable pulse oximetry waveform that measures oxygen saturation (SpO_2), however, serves as an accurate surrogate for the partial pressure of arterial oxygen (PaO_2) with a couple of notable exceptions—a pulse oximeter will be inaccurate during carbon monoxide poisoning and methemoglobinemia. Generally, the pulse oximeter allows for clinical predictions regarding severity of oxygen derangements without an ABG.[23] As a general guide, SpO_2 normally predicts PaO_2 based on the standard oxygen-hemoglobin dissociation curve (Table 1).

SpO2 (%)	PaO2 (mm Hg)
60	30
75	40
90	60
100	90

Table 1: Predicted arterial partial pressure of oxygen (PaO2) based on oxygen saturation from pulse oximetry (SpO2). Values based on the standard oxygen-hemoglobin dissociation curve.

For nearly all presenters to the emergency department, minimal differences exist between arterial and venous blood samples with respect to pH, HCO_3^-, and lactate. Several studies have demonstrated a strong correlation between arterial and venous pH across a range of conditions including respiratory compromise such as obstructive pulmonary disease and metabolic derangements such as diabetic ketoacidosis, with a mean pH difference of 0.03–0.04.[22–29]

The data surrounding blood gas sampling in patients with circulatory failure is conflicting. At least one study demonstrates good correlation between arterial and venous measurements of pH, HCO_3^-, and lactate across a range of blood pressures,[30] but others have demonstrated discrepancies.[19,20] The possible lack of correlation highlights the usefulness of obtaining venous sampling to determine tissue pH rather than an ABG.[19]

It should be noted that some of the referenced studies use central or mixed venous blood gas sampling as opposed to peripheral—a modality almost never immediately available to emergency physicians. For the most critically ill patients in circulatory compromise, the most complete physiology picture is determined using both central venous and arterial measurements. However, for the overwhelming majority of patients presenting to the emergency department with metabolic and/or respiratory illnesses, peripheral venous samples are adequate when combined with data from pulse oximetry, and management is rarely changed by obtaining arterial samples.[23,31]

As a bonus, when the pulse oximeter reading is in doubt (i.e. from a poisoning), many blood gas instruments perform co-oximetry, which differentiates oxyhemoglobin from methemoglobin, carboxyhemoglobin, and deoxyhemoglobin.[32] This allows for diagnosis of CO poisoning and methemoglobinemia without needing an ABG. For CO levels < 20% arterial and venous blood samples correlate nearly perfectly.[33]

The Bottom Line

- For most emergency department and critically ill patients, a venous blood gas can be used in place of an arterial blood gas for clinical decision making.

- A venous blood gas accurately reflects pH, HCO_3^-, and lactate with clinically insignificant differences from arterial samples.

- Severe circulatory compromise can create disparities between arterial and venous samples, but venous samples more accurately reflect the true tissue pH.

- Venous samples are sensitive to rule out hypercarbia when $pCO_2 < 45$ mmHg.

- Oxygenation status is often accurately assessed by pulse oximetry.

Backboards provide spinal immobilization

Daniel G. Ostermayer

The Origin

Backboards were initially adopted as a means of moving a dead or severely wounded patient during field trauma care. Eventually, wooden boards such as the Parr Backboard and Henley Board gave way to plastic or aluminum easy-to-clean long boards. Many EMS agencies allow for stay-on-the-board during hospital transport. This pattern of remaining on the board after extrication until "spinal clearance" by an emergency physician most likely created the misperception that the backboard provides spinal immobilization.

The Facts

No randomized trials for spinal immobilization exist but other studies in patients without injuries provide insights into the futility of the long board for spinal immobilization. Cervical spine immobilization, which is addressed in a separate chapter, has no relation to backboard management (cervical spine injuries are generally managed with a cervical collar regardless of the presence of a backboard). Also, without appropriate occipital padding on a backboard, neutral cervical positioning cannot be maintained.[34]

Injuries to the thoracic and lumbar spinal column are exceedingly rare in the setting of motor vehicle accidents.[35] Even if a fracture were present, the backboard provides little immobilization compared to a standard stretcher. A study of nine healthy volunteers without any back injuries randomized participants to immobilization on a long back board or a stretcher mattress while wearing a cervical collar; they were then driven through a road course to simulate hospital transport. The degree of lateral spine movement was assessed to determine if the backboard had provided any immobilization during transport. Mean lateral movement on the backboard was 2.22 cm for the chest (compared to 1.22 cm on the stretcher) and 1.88 cm at the hips (compared to 1.2 cm on the stretcher). The study also found that the greater the BMI the greater the degree of movement on a backboard.[36]

Although the backboard assists operationally during extrication, it may have a *negative* impact on cervical spine immobilization. In simulated patient extrications from automobiles, 3D motion analysis found no cervical spine movement reduction when a patient was on a backboard even with a c-collar in place.[37]

When patients in two prehospital systems (New Mexico and Malaysia) were compared, despite the fact that the Malaysian system did not use cervical collars or backboards, no differences in neurologic disability were found. Both groups of patients had cervical, thoracic or lumbosacral injuries. The similarity in outcomes between these disparate trauma systems could have resulted from unidentified confounders, but is equally likely due to the lack of true immobilization provided by backboards in the U.S.

system, or even due to the difficulty (perhaps impossibility) of providing spinal immobilization, regardless of method, in the prehospital environment.[38]

Backboard immobilization also causes pain and patient agitation, and increases the risk of respiratory compromise in the critically ill.[39] In healthy patients, lying on a long board for 30 minutes begins to cause sacral tissue ischemia and can produce pressure ulcers.[40] No evidence supports using a backboard as an immobilization device.

The Bottom Line

- Backboards do not immobilize the thoracic or lumbar spine.
- Immobilization and transport on backboards increase patients' risks for pain, tissue ischemia, respiratory impairment, and agitation.
- Long or short backboards can assist with patient extrication but do not provide immobilization during extrication.

A radial pulse indicates a systolic blood pressure of at least 80 mmHg

Tom Fadial, Daniel G. Ostermayer

The Origin

Rapidly estimating systolic blood pressure has obvious benefits, potentially guiding early escalation of therapy in critically ill patients. A proposed correlation between the presence of a palpable arterial pulse at specific central and peripheral arterial sites has a mysterious origin. The earliest Advanced Trauma Life Support (ATLS) course manuals taught palpation of the carotid, femoral, and then radial arteries to determine increasing systolic blood pressures.[41]

Site	Estimated Blood Pressure (mmHg)
Radial	>80
Femoral	70-80
Carotid	60-70

The Facts

This heuristic for estimating blood pressure was first challenged by Poulton in 1988 in an analysis of twenty trauma patients with noninvasive blood pressure measurements of less than 90 mmHg. Though a description of the methods and analysis was limited, Poulton found that the ATLS grading was accurate in only 25% of cases. More importantly, the study suggested blood pressure frequently overestimated the noninvasive measurement—particularly when blood pressure was lowest.[42]

In 2000, Deakin et al. expanded on the prior study in twenty patients with hypovolemic shock (etiology not specified). While the study supported the physiologically-sound notion that distal perfusion would dissipate prior to central pulsations (radial, then femoral, then carotid), they found that approximation by pulse palpation overestimated the gold standard—in this case invasive arterial blood pressure monitoring. The minimum blood pressure predicted by the guidelines was exceeded in only 4 of 20 patients, with the others less than predicted by palpation.[43]

Valuable data can be collected from the presence (and even quality)[44] of arterial pulsations on trauma primary survey and during the initial resuscitation of critically ill patients. However, the literature does not support using these pulsations to estimate a specific blood pressure range. The identification of even transient hypotension in trauma patients is of critical importance, warranting the activation of additional resources (surgical consultation, massive blood product transfusion, etc.). In specific injury settings, hypotension prompts immediate operative management (abdominal trauma with intraperitoneal hemorrhage) and portends ominous consequences (increased morbidity for traumatic brain injury[45]). Relying on this inaccurate heuristic, especially as it appears to lead to overestimation, could lead to inappropriate decision-making and should be avoided if invasive or noninvasive measurements are available.[46]

The Bottom Line

- Correlating a specific blood pressure to the location of a palpable pulse does not provide an accurate interpretation of blood pressure.
- Blood pressure is most likely overestimated by site specific palpation.
- Providers, especially in the prehospital environment, should n base resuscitation decisions on blood pressure estimation by palpation.

Non-steroidal anti-inflammatory medications decrease bone healing

John R. Ayers, Benjamin L. Cooper

The Origin

Non-steroidal anti-inflammatory drugs (NSAIDs) have been used to control acute pain for millennia. The first recorded use around 400 B.C. occurred when Hippocrates administered extract of willow (active ingredient salicin) bark to relieve pain.[47] Aspirin's mechanism of action remained unknown until the 1970s when John Vane discovered its inhibition of the production of prostaglandins, the product of an enzyme cyclooxygenase or COX.[48] Several other medications such as indomethacin were then synthesized with mechanisms of action similar to aspirin's and together form the broad class known as non-steroidal anti-inflammatory drugs (NSAIDs).

Concern over NSAIDs' effect on bone development began in the 1990s when multiple in vitro and animal studies demonstrated the importance of prostaglandins in bone development. This discovery fueled a concern that NSAIDs could negatively impact bone healing after a fracture—a concern compounded in pediatric patients whose bones are still developing.[49,50]

The Facts

Multiple studies confirm the importance of prostaglandins in bone healing. One demonstrated that fracture healing and bone formation was impaired in COX-2 null mice.[51] Given the potential risk of impaired bone healing, physicians became skeptical about the use of NSAIDs in acute fractures. NSAIDs, however, offer some of the most effective analgesia for acute musculoskeletal pain; several recent studies suggest that this class of drugs is at least as effective as opioids—if not more so—for relieving acute extremity pain.[52,53] NSAIDs also are not associated with the risk of respiratory depression or substance use disorder—important considerations given the effects of current opioid epidemics.

Retrospective studies have failed to consistently demonstrate increased rates of nonunion associated with NSAID use, and no convincing evidence exists that a short course of NSAIDs adversely affects bone healing.[54] Two randomized controlled trials (RCTs) of patients with distal radius fractures failed to demonstrate an effect of NSAIDs on the rate of bone healing or functional recovery after 2 and 4 weeks of exposure.[55] Two additional RCTs found prolonged (6 weeks) indomethacin use increased rates of nonunion in acetabular fractures. These studies suggest that the risk of nonunion may be related to both the duration of exposure and the dose.[56,57] In pediatric patients, two retrospective reviews found no difference in complication rates (including nonunion) when patients were exposed to ketorolac or ibuprofen. Details on dosing, however, were not reported, severely limiting generalizability.[58,59]

Several systematic reviews and one meta-analysis agree that there is no clear evidence that NSAIDs delay healing, and when higher quality studies are considered, there is no statistically significant association between NSAID exposure and nonunion.[48,54,60,61] By contrast, other factors have consistently been identified as risks for delayed healing—age, body mass index, smoking, alcohol consumption, comorbidities, and malnutrition.[54] A short course (1-2 weeks) of NSAIDs for acute pain related to an extremity fracture is unlikely to adversely affect healing.

The Bottom Line

- NSAIDs inhibit prostaglandin production via cyclooxygenase.
- Prostaglandins have a role in bone development, and inhibition of prostaglandin production could theoretically disrupt bone fracture healing.
- Retrospective studies show no association between NSAIDs and nonunion in pediatric patients, and RCTs have failed to demonstrate an effect of NSAIDs on bone fracture healing.
- NSAIDs are a very effective mode of analgesia and short courses, both prescribed and intermittently dosed in the emergency department, can help treat fracture-related pain.

Squamous cells in a urine sample indicate contamination and therefore prevent interpretation

Daniel. G. Ostermayer

The Origin

Leading medical and emergency medicine textbooks have taught that the presence of squamous epithelial cells (SECs) in urine specimen indicates contamination and prevents accurate interpretation of a urinary tract infection. Since squamous cells i the urine originate from the distal urethra or vulvovaginal region their presence implies inadequate perineal cleaning. Inadequate cleaning results in contamination and inaccurate determination the presence or absence of a urinary tract infection.

The Facts

Two studies performed in the emergency department provide evidence against SECs indicating gross contamination, but do raise questions about the accuracy of the urinalysis results in th presence of many SECs. The first, by Walter et al., prospectivel sampled 105 women in the emergency department with symptoms of a urinary tract infection (UTI).[62] A midstream clean catch and a catheterized urinalysis were performed on all patier with a possible UTI. The second study, a retrospective cross sectional analysis by Mohr et al., improved on the sample size c the original study by including 19,328 patients with a urinalysis performed.[63] Both studies used the common definition of a positive urine culture as $>10^4$/mL of gram-negative organisms or $>10^5$/mL gram-positive organisms. Contaminated samples were those growing mixed flora or non-urinary pathogens. Mohr's study also defined a positive urinalysis as >5 WBCs/mL with positive nitrites.[64]

Walter et al. found SECs in 95% of the catheter specimens but no urinary contamination. In the midstream catch specimens, 96% contained SECs but only 21% were contaminated. This highlights the fact that SECs are very common in urine specimens but don't necessarily indicate contamination with non-urine-originating bacteria.[62] SECs, however, do impact the performance characteristics of the urinalysis because of an associated WBC increase. Often, the greater the number of SECs the greater the degree of pyuria due to labial WBCs entering the urinary sample along with the SECs. This false increase in pyuria is not associated with an increase in the presence of nitrites. This equates to a distortion of the accuracy of a positive urinalysis based on WBC and leukocyte esterase positivity when significant SECs are present.

If greater than 8 SECs/high powered field (hpf) are present in the urine sample and the results indicate a urinary tract infection, a new clean catch or catheterized sample is needed. The likelihood ratio of a positive urinalysis predicting a culture positive UTI with >8 SECs/hpf decreases from 4.98 (moderately useful) to 2.35 (not useful).[63,65] However, a negative urinalysis can still be relied upon regardless of SEC positivity. If a urinalysis is negative, then the test can still assist with ruling out a UTI since the negative likelihood ratios are not affected by the presence o SECs.[62,63,65] A positive urinalysis in the presence of >8 SECs/hr should be repeated for a cleaner sample if positive is based onl' on WBC criteria. If nitrite-positive, a new sample is not necessai

The Bottom Line

- SECs do not affect culture results or predict bacterial urine specimen contamination.
- False positive urinalysis results due to increased pyuria can occur in samples with SECs due to labial and vaginal WBCs.
- Nitrite results should not be affected by SEC presence.
- A negative urinalysis regardless of SEC presence can be interpreted as negative.

High dose rocuronium provides equivalent speed to paralysis as succinylcholine

Daniel G. Ostermayer

The Origin

Concerns about the contraindications of succinylcholine coupled with the recently available reversal medication for rocuronium, sugammadex, have caused wide spread adoption of rocuronium in the ED under the impression that high doses (1.2 mg/kg) create equivalent intubation conditions and speed of paralysis.[66] High dose rocuronium is reported to have an equal time to paralysis as succinylcholine with the added benefits of a long duration without the adverse effects that theoretically plague succinylcholine. Specifically, succinylcholine can elevate (approximately 0.5 mEq/L) serum potassium in all patients, potentially much higher with chronic denervation (previous burns, severe crush injuries or neuromuscular diseases),[67] and can induce malignant hyperthermia in predisposed patients.[68]

The Facts

Two often cited studies describe equivalent intubating conditions for rocuronium and succinylcholine comparing usage in the operating room[69], and extracting retrospective comparison from an emergency department chart review.[70] Both studies may have lacked sufficient power to detect superiority among the paralytics, but do provide insights into pragmatic usage. In the operating-room study,[69] a time frame of up to 60 seconds was established to wait for optimal intubating conditions when comparing paralytics, which may be appropriate for elective intubations with healthy physiology and ideal preoxygenation, b not for critical patients. Succinylcholine (1.5 mg/kg) has a time t paralysis of 34s compared to rocuronium's 54s (at 1.2mg/kg dosing).[71] This additional 20 seconds to obtain adequate paralysis could equate to a clinically significant impact in the critically ill patient when intubating conditions are not ideal.

A meta-analysis of randomized controlled trials comparing rocuronium vs succinylcholine for rapid sequence induction, an secondary analysis of only those with high-dose paralytic use (mg/kg of succinylcholine and 1.2 mg/kg of rocuronium), report 84% excellent intubating conditions in succinylcholine versus 66% with rocuronium.[72] This is most likely due to the speed of onset, where time to paralysis produces the greatest impact on success. A second meta-analysis, with additional tria added in 2015, produced the same conclusion—that intubating conditions are superior when using succinylcholine—and additionally stated that rocuronium should only be used if a contraindication exists to succinylcholine administration.[73]

The Bottom Line

- High dose rocuronium dosing produces a speed of onset that on average 20 seconds slower than succinylcholine.
- The delay in paralysis with 1.2 mg/kg of rocuronium produces excellent intubating conditions less often than 1.5 mg/kg of succinylcholine.

Topical anesthetics are unsafe for corneal abrasions

Benjamin L. Cooper

The Origin

Acute pain due to corneal abrasions represent a large portion of eye-related injuries presenting to the emergency department. The pain from a corneal abrasion can be severe and can result in disrupted daily function, missed work, and lost sleep. Traditional measures to control pain include topical and oral non-steroidal anti-inflammatory agents and cycloplegics. In the past, corneal abrasions were treated with eye patching, which provides no improvement in pain while potentially increasing risk of infection.[74] Application of a topical ocular anesthetic provides immediate pain relief from corneal abrasions—a virtually diagnostic maneuver—but concern about corneal toxicity has limited their use in the outpatient setting. For decades, textbooks have consistently cited the toxic effects of topical anesthetics and discouraged their use for cornea-related pain. Adverse events reported in widely cited case series include corneal ulcerations, keratitis, and rare candida co-infection.[75,76] Proposed mechanisms for toxicity include suppression of self-protective reflexes and tearing as well as direct cytotoxic effects.[77–81]

The Facts

Most of the literature stigmatizing the use of topical anesthetics stems from animal studies and from case reports of topical anesthetic *abuse,* not controlled prescribed use. An emerging body of literature supports the *limited* use of topical anesthetics for corneal abrasions.[77–81] Several publications from the ophthalmology literature report the safety of outpatient use of dilute anesthetics after photorefractive surgery.[81] At the time of this writing, three double-blind randomized controlled trials conducted in the emergency department have evaluated the safety and efficacy of topical anesthetics for simple corneal abrasions, and all concluded no increased risk of adverse even or delayed healing related to topical anesthetic use.[78–80]

All trials excluded complicated features like delayed presentation (>36 hours), presence of rust ring, infection, previous eye injury or complicating pathology (retinopathy or glaucoma), and all were given topical antibiotics for infection prevention. The anesthetic concentrations, and instructions for use were as follows: 1 drop of tetracaine 0.4% applied hourly a needed for 48 hours,[78] 1 drop of tetracaine 1% applied every 3(minutes as needed for up to 48 hours,[80] and 2-4 drops of dilute proparacaine 0.05% as needed (without dosing interval specifie for up to 7 days.[79] These studies were small (total n = 196) and adverse event rates were low with no reported serious adverse events (e.g. ulcerations or coinfections). A larger, more recent observational study of 532 patients with simple corneal abrasio reported no serious complications or adverse events attributed topical use of tetracaine.[81]

The Bottom Line

- Case reports originally suggested topical anesthetic abuse is associated with corneal toxicity and may result in adverse events.
- An emerging body of literature is supportive of limited use (<48 hours) of dilute topical anesthetics for simple corneal abrasions.
- Topical anesthetic preparation options for short-term use include 1 drop of tetracaine 1% applied every 30 minutes as needed, and 2-4 drops of dilute proparacaine 0.05% as needed

Blood pressure control assists with bleeding cessation during epistaxis

Benjamin L. Cooper, Daniel G. Ostermayer

The Origin

Several local and systemic factors appear to contribute to epistaxis regardless of whether the source of bleeding is located anteriorly (Kiesselbach's plexus) or posteriorly (sphenopalatine artery). Local factors include digital trauma (i.e. nose-picking), mucosal trauma, nasal administered drugs, dehumidification from cold and dry climates, and rhinitis. Systemic bleeding disorders drug-induced or otherwise, and hereditary conditions (e.g. hereditary telangiectasia) also contribute.[82] The contribution of high blood pressure to epistaxis, however, has long been debated.[83]

The origin dates to a 1930s publication describing arterial hypertension and the occurrence of epistaxis.[84] Physiologically patients with chronic hypertension may have micro-vascular damage that increases their risk of epistaxis,[85] or the epistaxis itself may induce the hypertensive event. Traditional teaching has encouraged acute blood pressure control alongside hemostatic techniques[82] to both reduce incidence and control bleeding.

The Facts

Two studies demonstrated a lack of association between hypertension and epistaxis.[86,87] The largest, a population-based study of 1174 people in Brazil, could not demonstrate an association when controlling for multiple factors such as age, gender, abuse of alcohol, history of allergic rhinitis, and nasal abnormalities. While two studies demonstrate a lack of association between hypertension and epistaxis, systematic reviews and meta-analyses suggest a positive association. The meta-analyses, however, contain significant heterogeneity, limiting interpretation. Without randomized controlled trials to evaluate the effect of blood pressure management on recurrent epistaxis, the available data is subject to confounding.[83,88]

An ED study of patients with persistent epistaxis on admission found an association with a medical history of hypertension and a small difference in admission systolic blood pressure (166 vs 153 mmHg).[89] A prospective matched case-control study in the ED found patients with epistaxis to have greater systolic blood pressures (161 vs 144 mmHg) than matched patients without epistaxis.[90] These and many other small studies suggest association, not causation.[83,91,92]

At the time of this writing, there are still no published RCTs to evaluate the effect of blood pressure management, acute or chronic, on recurrent epistaxis. It is difficult to determine if hypertension is the cause of an acute episode of epistaxis since many patients will have consequent and co-presenting anxiety, and many people with comorbidities such as hypertension will have a greater risk for epistaxis that is not digital trauma related.[82] Also, application of common vasoconstrictors such as phenylephrine or oxymetazoline can cause blood pressure elevation during treatment. As previously stated, the association of hypertension and epistaxis should not be interpreted as causation.

The mainstay of treatment for epistaxis remains source contr via one or more of the mechanisms available in clinical practice.[93–95] *After* adequate control of the patient's symptoms and serial blood pressure measurements, the consideration of blood pressure management may be reasonable, but should nc be a first line intervention.

The Bottom Line

- Hypertension is associated with epistaxis, but causation has n been demonstrated.
- Blood pressure control should not be included in the initial goa of managing acute epistaxis due to the importance of establishing source control.
- First line techniques for hemostasis should include topical vasoconstriction, pressure application, and clot stabilization.

Cervical collars are necessary to prevent cervical spine injury following blunt trauma

Nikhil R. Patel, Daniel G. Ostermayer

The Origin

Cervical spinal (c-spine) immobilization following blunt trauma began with the use of sandbags and tape for immobilization during the Vietnam War, before being formally adopted into the early ATLS protocols.[96,97] Because of early estimates that up to 25% of cervical spine trauma resulted from improper immobilization status post-injury, cervical collars (c-collars) and c-spine precautions became ingrained in the practice of ATLS without a solid evidence base.[98,99]

The Facts

The benefit imputed to c-collars in acute trauma hinges on their effectively reducing range of motion (ROM) and reducing the incidence of neurologic injuries that result from improper immobilization. C-collars do not prevent further boney injury but instead aim to prevent cord injury by reducing mobility in the setting of a possibly unstable fracture. Podolsky et al. published one of the initial studies using various c-spine immobilization techniques like the traditional tape and sandbag method and a series of collars (soft, hard, extrication, Philadelphia) on twenty-five healthy volunteers. Without c-collar immobilization the participants had a baseline ROM of 36° of flexion, 21° extension, 21° lateral movement, and 76° rotation.[98] The sandbags with tape demonstrated superiority in motion restriction with respectively 0.1°, 15°, 1.8°, and 2.5° of motion compared to the Philadelphia collar's 24.2°, 12°, 17.4°, and 49.9° of motion. Sandbags used in conjunction with c-collars reduced movement to as little as 0.1°, 7.4°, 1.4°, and 4.0° of motion.[98]

Based upon the described core range of motion study, c-collars became standard-of-care for blunt trauma patients, potentially limiting further study in randomized trials. A 2001 Cochrane Review found no randomized controlled trials (RCTs) of spinal immobilization strategies in trauma patients.[99] A 2011 cadaveric study measured ROM of the neck with both stable and unstable fractures after a c-collar had been placed by an orthopedist, finding equivocal ROM for one-piece collars, two-piece collars, and no collars.[100] A 2012 trial of sixteen healthy participants in a simulated car extrication compared four immobilization techniques—uncollared while self-extricating, collared while self-extricating, collared with assisted extrication, and collared while on an extrication device. Three-dimensional (3D) trackers demonstrated motion reduction by 20° with the c-collar while the patient self-extricated. Placing the patient on a backboard or Kendrick Extrication Device did not further restrict ROM.[37] Similar studies observed 6.6° of head movement for a collared patient self-extricating.[7] The average ROM for an uncollared patient self-extricating was 13.33°.[101]

Although the c-collar does limit range of motion, their clinical utility was questioned by a 1998 landmark study.[99] This five-year retrospective study compared 334 New Mexican and 120 Malaysian patients with similar blunt traumatic injuries. The New Mexican patients had c-collars placed as a matter of routine compared to none of the Malaysian patients. When the odds ratios for any post-traumatic neurologic injury between collared (U.S.) and un-collared (Malaysian) patients were compared, it was found that patients wearing c-collars had an odds ratio for clinical disability of 2.03 for the whole cervical spine and 1.52 for any individual level. The authors estimated that "the probability of finding data as extreme as this if immobilization has an overall beneficial effect is only 2%." In other words, c-collars have a 98% chance of being at best useless and may be potentially harmful.[38]

Adverse effects of c-collars include pain, ulceration, exacerbated injury if improperly sized, increased intracranial pressure, worsening respiratory status, increased aspiration risk, compromised airway management, delayed transport, delayed resuscitation, delayed definitive care, and missed injuries.[102] Also, a cadaveric study demonstrated that application of a c-collar increased the distance between C1 and C2 by as much as 7.3 mm in the presence of an unstable fracture.[103] Given the possibility of harm and lacking evidence of clinical benefit, the range of motion restriction provided by prehospital c-collars has questionable benefit. The American Association for Neurological Surgeons and Congress of Neurological Surgeons recommend c-collar use for nonverbal, obtunded, neurologically injured patients, and for blunt trauma patients with severe mechanisms of injury. Fully awake, non-intoxicated, communicating patients without neck tenderness, neurologic abnormality or distracting injury should not be immobilized.[104]

The Bottom Line

- Cervical spine collars do decrease range of motion of the cervical spine but if applied or sized improperly may worsen an unstable injury.
- No patient-centered clinical benefit from cervical collar placement has been demonstrated.
- Multiple adverse effects may result from cervical collars with both immediate and prolonged use.
- No specific range of motion limitation has been associated with cervical spine injury prevention.
- Head blocks or sandbags and tape immobilize more effectively than any c-collar.
- Routine use of c-collars in trauma patients is not supported by the current evidence.

"Stone heart" occurs when IV calcium is administered to a patient with digoxin toxicity

Benjamin L. Cooper, John C. Waller-Delarosa

The Origin

Digoxin is a cardiac glycoside that simultaneously increases contractility and slows atrioventricular conduction by inhibiting the Na^+/K^+ ATPase pump exchanger. Botanically derived, it was discovered over a century ago. It has the net effect of increasing extracellular potassium and increasing intracellular calcium. Digoxin toxicity manifests with multisystem symptoms including gastrointestinal (nausea/vomiting/diarrhea), cardiac dysrhythmias (partial depolarization of the myocardium leads to an excitable state), and visual aberrations. Therapy for digoxin toxicity includes treatment of life-threatening arrhythmias and neutralization of digoxin with digoxin-binding antibodies.[105]

With acute digoxin toxicity, the increase in extracellular potassium could potentially lead to dysrhythmias. There exists a longstanding belief that temporization of the cardiac membrane under conditions of hyperkalemia with intravenous calcium could induce a "stone heart" by causing even greater increases in intracellular calcium. The administration of IV calcium could impair cardiac relaxation and induce tetany—hence the name "stone heart."[106]

This theory seems to originate from several sources. First, animal studies in the early 1930s reported that prior "sensitization" with large doses of calcium appeared to lower the toxic threshold of cardiac glycosides.[107,108] Second, a 1936 case series reported on two post-operative patients on several days of therapy with "digalen" (a purified digitalis preparation last available 1964) who died shortly after administration of IV calcium.[106,108] This led to the dogmatic belief that calcium administration is contraindicated in digoxin toxicity. Further perpetuating this notion, another 1957 publication evaluating digitalis toxicity described two patients who were "fully digitalized" then died after IV calcium administration.[106,109]

The Facts

Since the original literature was published, many articles have questioned the validity of the "stone heart" theory. The methodologies of the original literature do not stand up to modern scrutiny, often describing cases subject to extensive confounding and with key information absent (such as digoxin levels, potassium levels, and calcium levels).[106,107] Multiple modern animal studies contradict earlier suggestions of calcium-digoxin synergy except for when near-toxic levels of serum calcium were induced.[107,110] A randomized controlled animal trial in which digoxin toxicity was induced, and subsequent hyperkalemia treated with either IV calcium or placebo, demonstrated no harm from calcium administration.[111] Several case reports have been published examining patients with hyperkalemia treated with calcium without ill effects despite supratherapeutic digoxin levels.[112,113] Most recently, a 2011 retrospective chart review identifying 159 patients with digoxin toxicity found no difference mortality between the groups of those given calcium and those from whom it was withheld.[106]

The Bottom Line

- Digoxin has a narrow therapeutic window and can cause several cardiac dysrhythmias.
- The original case reports of "stone heart" contain methodological flaws and are inconsistent with modern case series.
- The "stone heart" theory of IV calcium use in the setting of digoxin toxicity is unlikely to be true especially at therapeutic doses of calcium used for treating hyperkalemia.
- When the ECG shows signs of hyperkalemia in the setting of acute digoxin poisoning, IV calcium should be administered.

Epinephrine use during cardiac arrest improves patient outcomes

Benjamin L. Cooper, Richard B. Witkov

The Origin

The administration of epinephrine is a core part of advanced life support algorithms for cardiac arrest care. Epinephrine's origin can be traced to the late 1800s and early 1900s, when adrenal extracts were used to revive isolated animal hearts; subsequent experimentation in animal models culminated in the synthesis of epinephrine in 1905. In 1906, Crile and Dolley demonstrated that infusion of epinephrine improved successful resuscitation rates in dogs when compared with artificial ventilation and cardiac massage alone.[114] The mechanism behind epinephrine's efficacy at increasing the return of spontaneous circulation (ROSC) after cardiac arrest predominantly involves its effect on alpha-1 receptor stimulation of vascular smooth muscle. This induces vasoconstriction which in turn increases aortic diastolic pressure, leading to increased coronary perfusion pressure and cerebral perfusion pressure.[115]

Per the American Heart Association 2015 guidelines, "standard-dose epinephrine (1 mg every 3 to 5 minutes) may be reasonable for patients in cardiac arrest" (a Class IIb [weak] recommendation).[116]

The Facts

Epinephrine utilization may result in increased tachydysrhythmias, increased myocardial oxygen demand, and reduced microvascular perfusion, all of which are undesirable effects in the cardiac arrest patient.[115] Most clinical data on epinephrine use is observational and derived from the All-Japan out-of-hospital cardiac arrest (OHCA) registry. Two major studies evaluated a subset of OHCA patients with a shockable rhythm, and the results were conflicting. In both studies epinephrine use was associated with lower rates of ROSC (21.6% vs 28.1%; 22.8% vs 27.7%), one-month survival (16.5% vs 28.8%; 15.4 vs 27.0%), and neurologically intact survival (6.9% vs 19.8%; 7.0% vs 18.6%); when using a propensity-score matched model to adjust for covariates in one of the studies, the odds of one-month survival were greater for those receiving epinephrine (adjusted odds ratio [aOR] 1.34, 95% confidence interval [CI] 1.12-1.60), *but there was no difference in the odds of neurologically intact survival* (aOR 1.01, 95% CI 0.78-1.30).

For non-shockable rhythms, both studies report epinephrine use as associated with higher rates of ROSC (18.5% vs 5.7%, and 18.7% vs 3.0%) and one-month survival in the adjusted analysis, while one study found slightly higher odds of neurologically intact survival (aOR 1.57, 95% CI 1.04-2.37).[117,118] The largest observational study included OHCA patients and did not perform subgroup analysis based on shockable vs non-shockable rhythms. This study reported increased ROSC with epinephrine use (18.5% vs 15.7%), decreased one-month survival (aOR 0.54, 95% CI 0.43-0.68), and decreased neurologically intact survival (1.4% vs 2.2%, aOR 0.21, 95% CI 0.10-0.44).[119] The results of these studies are summarized in Table 1.

Table 1. Summary of outcome data from the Japan OHCA registry.

Author	Hagihara	Nakahara	Goto	Goto	Nakahara
Period	2005-2008	2007-2010	2009-2010	2009-2010	2007-2010
Subset	NA	Shockable	Shockable	Non-shockable	Non-shockable
Number of cases	417,188	14,943	15,492	194,085	81,136
ROSC with epi[a]	18.5%	21.6%	22.8%	18.7%	18.5%
ROSC w/o epi[a]	5.7%	28.1%	27.7%	3.0%	5.7%
aOR (95% CI)	3.75 (3.59-3.91)[c]	NA	1.45 (1.20-1.75)[e]	8.83 (8.01-9.73)[e]	NA
1-mo survival with epi[a]	5.4%	16.5%	15.4%	3.9%	3.9%
1-mo survival w/o epi[a]	4.7%	28.8%	27.0%	2.2%	4.2%
aOR (95% CI)	0.54 (0.43-0.68)[c]	1.34 (1.12-1.60)[d]	0.95 (0.77-1.16)[e]	1.78 (1.5-2.10)[e]	1.72 (1.45-2.04)[d]
CPC[b] 1-2 with epi[a]	1.4%	6.9%	7.0%	0.59%	0.6%
CPC[b] 1-2 w/o epi[a]	2.2%	19.8%	18.6%	0.62%	1.5%
aOR (95% CI)	0.21 (0.10-0.44)[c]	1.01 (0.78-1.30)[d]	0.71 (0.54-0.92)[e]	0.95 (0.62-1.37)[e]	1.57 (1.04-2.37)[d]

[a]Epinephrine. [b]Cerebral Performance Category (category 1, good cerebral performance; category 2, moderate cerebral disability; category 3, severe cerebral disability; category 4, coma or vegetative state; category 5, death). [c]Data adjusted for propensity and all covariates. [d]Time-dependent propensity-score matched data. [e]Epinephrine given within 9 minutes; data adjusted via logistic regression.

A recent meta-analysis of 14 studies with 655,853 patients concluded that while epinephrine increased ROSC, its use doe not increase survival to discharge and increases the likelihood that discharged patients will have a poor neurologic outcome.[12] The observational nature of these initial studies predisposes th to significant confounding, necessitating investigation via RCT.

Prior to 2018, there were two RCTs that evaluated the effect epinephrine. In a Norwegian study, 851 OHCA patients were randomized to receive intravenous access and drugs as indica or IV access delayed until 5 minutes after ROSC. Among those with a shockable rhythm, there was no difference in rates of ROSC, survival to admission, or survival to discharge. Among those with a non-shockable rhythm, higher rates of ROSC (29% vs 11%) and survival to admission (19% vs 10%) were achieve in the IV access group, but not survival to discharge (2% vs 3%).[121] Another RCT from Western Australia randomized 534 OHCA patients to receive epinephrine vs placebo. For shockat rhythms the response to epinephrine was favorable for ROSC (26.9% vs 13.5%) and survival to admission (27.7% vs 15.1%) but not statistically significant for survival to discharge . For no shockable rhythms, patients receiving epinephrine showed markedly higher rates of ROSC (20.9% vs 3.7%) and survival admission (23.5% vs 11%), but not survival to discharge.

In 2018, Perkins et al. published "A Randomized Trial of Epinephrine in Out-of-Hospital Cardiac Arrest," also known as PARAMEDIC-2 trial, analyzing epinephrine use in out-of-hosp cardiac arrest. PARAMEDIC-2 is the third RCT evaluating the efficacy of epinephrine in cardiac arrest, and the largest to date. 8,014 patients with out-of-hospital cardiac arrest in the United Kingdom were randomized to receive epinephrine or saline placebo. The primary outcome was the rate of survival at 30 days, with a secondary outcome of rate of survival to hospital discharge with a favorable neurologic outcome. Overall, the use of epinephrine resulted in a significantly higher 30-day survival than placebo (3.2% vs 2.4%) without a significantly higher rate of favorable neurologic outcome (2.2% vs 1.9%).[122] Subgroup analyses were not included. Results from the 3 referenced RCTs are summarized in Table 2.

Table 2. Summary of outcomes from 3 RCTs evaluating the use of epinephrine in OHCA.

Author	Olasveengen	Jacobs	Jacobs	Olasveengen	Perki(n)
Period	2003-2008	2006-2009	2006-2009	2003-2008	2014-
Subset	Shockable	Shockable	Non-shockable	Non-shockable	NA
Total number of cases	286	245	289	565	8014
ROSC with epi[a]	59%	26.9%	20.9%	29%	36.3%
ROSC w/o epi[a]	53%	13.5%	3.7%	11%	11.7%
p-value	0.35	0.009	<.001	<.001	NA
Survival[b] with epi[a]	27%	7.6%	1.3%	2%	3.2%
Survival[b] w/o epi[a]	23%	4%	0%	3%	2.4%
p-value	0.45	0.23	NA	0.65	0.02
CPC[c] 1-2 with epi[a]	26%	Only two unfavorable neurologic outcomes occurred, and both were in the epinephrine group.		2%	2.2%[d]
CPC[c] 1-2 w/o epi[a]	20%			2%	1.9%[d]
p-value	0.36			0.82	OR 1. CI 0.8 1.61

[a]Epinephrine. [b]Survival to hospital discharge. [c]Cerebral Performance Category (category 1, good cerebral performance; category 2, moderate cerebral disability; category 3, severe cerebral disability; category 4, coma or vegetative state; category death). [d]Favorable neurologic outcome indicated by a score of 3 or less on the modi Rankin scale (ranges from 0 [no symptoms] to 6 [death]).

The Bottom Line

- Epinephrine utilization may result in increased tachydysrhythmias, increased myocardial oxygen demand, an reduced microvascular perfusion, all of which are undesirable effects in the cardiac arrest patient.

- Epinephrine helps to achieve return of spontaneous circulatio in patients with non-shockable rhythms.

- Epinephrine may help to achieve return of spontaneous circulation in patients with shockable rhythms, but at greatly diminished rates.

- Epinephrine appears to help achieve survival to hospital discharge in all patients with cardiac arrest, but with poorer neurologic outcomes.

The trauma "golden hour"

Christopher T. Stephens, Daniel G. Ostermayer

The Origin

The "golden hour" of trauma care is the age-old maxim that mortality increases significantly if definitive care and complete resuscitation do not occur within an hour of injury for patients w acute hemorrhage. While this concept has guided much of the modern approach to prehospital trauma resuscitation, many physicians have debated its scientific basis. The term "Golden Hour" originated at the University of Maryland hospital circa 19 and was most likely coined by Dr. R Adams Cowley. His team performed research at the first clinical shock trauma unit, know to those involved simply as the "death lab." Dr. Cowley, a fame heart surgeon turned trauma surgeon, was awarded a grant by the U.S. Army to study hemorrhagic shock. He and his team learned that they were able to resuscitate dogs suffering from hemorrhagic shock if they were able to intervene early,[123] and posited that perhaps similar means of time-based transfusions and hemorrhage control would translate to improved outcomes for trauma patients in Baltimore.

This study among many other canine experiments at Dr. Cowley's lab led to a belief that time contributed the greatest effect when resuscitating patients in hemorrhagic shock. As Cowley explained in an interview: "There is a golden hour between life and death. If you are critically injured, you have le than 60 minutes to survive. You might not die right then; it may three days or two weeks later...but something has happened in your body that is irreparable."[124]

Dogs that remained hypotensive from acute hemorrhage for greater than 60 minutes had a greater likelihood of death compared to those more rapidly transfused.[125] Physiologically, the "oxygen debt concept" served as a model for understanding how prolonged end-organ ischemia results from massive hemorrhage: when prolonged, hemorrhagic shock damages tissue to an extent that survival becomes impossible even if aggressive resuscitation strategies are implemented.[126] (Figure 1).

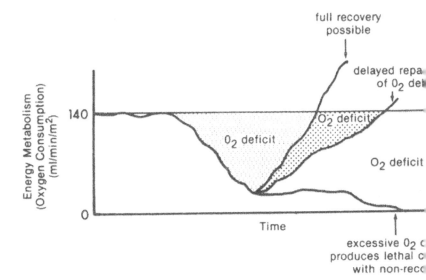

Figure 1. Oxygen debt curve[127]

The Facts

Unfortunately, no human studies have evaluated the precise "golden" window of time for hemorrhagic shock resuscitation. Although accepted as a matter of physiology that humans can only survive a shock state for so long, no data has supported or refuted the 60-minute time window. Military data suggests some truth to the Golden Hour. Trauma patient survival increased as time to definitive care decreased from 6 hours in prior wars to one hour during the Vietnam War. However, this dataset could not control for many other confounding factors such as advances in medical care beyond simply fast transport.[128] One small report from World War I in France suggests that patients treated within one hour of their injury had a mortality rate of 10%, with mortality increasing for each hour of delayed treatment to a 75% mortality rate after 8 hours.[129] Unfortunately military data may not directly translate to civilian care. Small civilian samples comparing trauma care in urban and rural regions suggest greater survival with shorter out of hospital times but cannot provide a definitive answer due to myriad confounders such as injury severity and destination capabilities.[130] Lerner and Moscati, performing a comprehensive review of the origins of the Golden Hour could not find any scientific justification for the term or study that specifically originated the phrasing.[131]

Despite the lack of human data to support the necessity of trauma resuscitation within 60 minutes, the Golden Hour is often applied to all patients with any traumatic injury. The term originated specifically in relation to hemorrhagic shock; even in that context, it remains unproven as a firm certain-mortality threshold that can guide clinical practice. In addition, the Golden Hour does not have any evidence or support for application in patients with non-shock-producing injuries.

Dr. Cowley took his idea to its logical conclusion by successfully campaigning for transport within 60 minutes, using helicopters as needed, from anywhere in the state to the University of Maryland Shock Trauma Center—establishing a trend. Intuition and operational experience support rapid intervention and transport to definitive care for trauma patients. Misinterpretation of the original Golden Hour, and unwarranted extrapolation from Cowley's hypothesis, could result in significant resource strain on tertiary care trauma centers.[132]

The Bottom Line

- Rapid resuscitation and transport to definitive care of trauma patients with severe hemorrhage has a strong physiologic basis.
- Prolonged hemorrhage deprives tissue of necessary oxygenation and may lead to irreversible cell death and greater mortality.
- No human data has supported or refuted the 60-minute time cutoff for hemorrhagic shock resuscitation.
- No operational data has refuted the idea that faster transport provides universally better trauma care.

The cremasteric reflex is absent during testicular torsion

Kian Preston-Suni, Ryan Pedigo

The Origin

John Hunter, in 1810, first reported a case of testicular torsion. A young man with two separate episodes of acute onset unilateral scrotal pain was treated with blood-letting and a warm compress of herbs, but unfortunately did not recover and had two atrophied testicles.[133] Then in 1894 Lauenstein described the underlying pathology of the disease[134], and later linked the similarities of clinical presentation with acute epididymitis, a much more benign condition. By the early 20th century, empiric surgical exploration of the acute scrotum was recommended in order to not miss testicular torsion since clinical exams could not accurately rule out the disease.[135]

Investigators throughout the last century have sought some reliable method to aid in diagnosis and avoid unnecessary surgeries. A published case series in 1984 provided the first evidence supporting the diagnostic utility of using the cremasteric reflex to rule out torsion. In a series of 245 boys with acute scrotal pain, all 56 patients with testicular torsion lacked a cremasteric reflex, while 66% of boys without torsion had an intact reflex.[136]

The Facts

Several published case series report the absence of the cremasteric reflex in all confirmed cases of testicular torsion.[137–]

[139] The cremasteric reflex, however, is frequently absent in other causes of acute scrotal pain. Caldemone et al. reported an absent cremasteric reflex in 25% of cases of acute epididymitis and 33% of cases of hydatid torsion (torsion of the appendix testis). Moreover, as many as 30% of normal asymptomatic patients fail to demonstrate a cremasteric reflex.[140] Even more concerning, a significant number of publications report an intact cremasteric reflex despite surgically confirmed torsion of the spermatic cord. The highest reported rate of intact cremasteric reflex in testicular torsion is by Van Glebke et al., who noted the reflex present in a striking 40% (10 of 25) of cases.[141] While no large prospective studies exist, many other case series report an intact cremasteric reflex in cases of confirmed testicular torsion, with rates ranging from 8% to 30%.[142–147] Therefore, the cremasteric reflex lacks reliability as a rule-in or rule-out test when evaluating a patient for possible testicular torsion.[148]

The Bottom Line

- The cremasteric reflex is often absent in normal testicles.
- Other causes of an acute scrotum may also have an absent cremasteric reflex.
- Testicular torsion may present with an intact cremasteric reflex.
- Presence of a cremasteric reflex cannot be used to rule out the diagnosis of testicular torsion, nor can its absence confirm torsion.

Atropine should be administered prior to succinylcholine during pediatric intubation

Irma T. Ugalde

The Origin

Pediatric resuscitation protocols such as Advanced Pediatric Life Support (APLS) and Pediatric Advanced Life Support (PALS) have recommended the use of 0.02 mg/kg atropine (minimum of 0.1 mg and maximum of 0.5 mg dose) before succinylcholine to prevent bradycardia and asystole in children prior to intubation.[149,150] These protocols and recommendations emerged from a publication in 1957 where Leigh and colleagues reported four cases of bradycardia in pediatric patients who received succinylcholine during rapid sequence intubation (RSI). The authors recommended routine use of atropine to prevent the bradycardia.[150] Then in 1960, a study demonstrated that after repeated doses of succinylcholine most of the 41 patients in the study developed a decrease in heart rate with two-thirds experiencing sinus bradycardia and the remainder with arrhythmias. The eleven patients with arrhythmias varied from p-wave abnormalities to QRS widening and ectopic beats to AV conduction dysfunction including ventricular standstill in seven of the eleven.[151] Five bradycardic patients received atropine prior to the next dose of succinylcholine and their heart rate increased to 100 beats/min. Green and coauthors reported heart rate changes in 26 anesthetized children with succinylcholine as the paralyzing agent and concluded that those receiving multiple doses of the agent should receive pre-treatment with an IV anticholinergic agent.[152]

The Facts

Both succinylcholine and laryngoscopy can induce bradycardia. Succinylcholine will act on vagal pathways and stimulate peripheral receptors which may induce a reflex bradycardia.[153] Intubation directly stimulates the pharynx, esophagus, and respiratory tract which may also cause a vasovagal reflex by stimulating the baroreceptor reflexes.[150,154] note, defecation, nasogastric tube placements, yawning, and hiccupping may also induce bradycardia or even intermittent respiratory pauses in infants, yet clinicians do not premedicate these procedures or conditions with atropine.[155]

Like bradycardia during defecation, the events during intubation have questionable clinical significance due to infant and neonatal physiology. Neonates and young infants have higher resting heart rates due to the greater sympathetic tone within their sinoatrial and atrioventricular nodes and less sympathetic innervation to the bundle branches and ventricles. These imbalances of the autonomic nervous system usually resolve by 6 to 9 months of age but prior to resolution cause exaggerated responses to stress.[156,157] Selective peripheral vasoconstriction compensates for any vagal reflex bradycardia order to maintain cerebral perfusion.[158]

To quantify the incidence of induced bradycardia beyond the initial case reports, McAuliffe et al. performed a single-blind randomized controlled trial where 41 surgical patients aged 1–12 received either atropine and succinylcholine or succinylcholine alone.[159] One bradycardic event and 7 dysrhythmias occurred in the atropine group compared to 0 and 3 in the succinylcholine only group. More recently, Fastle et al. examined 143 patients retrospectively between the ages of newborn to 19 years who underwent RSI, and compared the patients who did and did not receive atropine.[160] Three patients in each group experienced transient bradycardia. Only 4% of those who received rocuronium experienced an event which resolved without intervention or clinical adverse effects. Sixteen of 143 patients received succinylcholine only and none of them experienced bradycardia.[160] The predominant effect of a decline in heart rate produced few if any attributable clinical effects.

The current and best available evidence does not support the indiscriminate use of atropine for pediatric intubation. Although repeat administration of succinylcholine is often not necessary, if performed it may be reasonable to consider atropine. In the worst cases of hypoxemia-related bradycardia, atropine would have no effect unless oxygenation was improved.[161] Hypoxia plays a more critical role in unstable bradycardia during RSI, so optimizing successful intubation conditions with preoxygenation will mitigate occurrence. In addition, adding another drug to the already high stress situation of emergent intubation could increase risk for dosing errors or procedural errors. In infants, atropine is associated with ventricular arrhythmias and malignant hyperthermia.[162,163]

The Bottom Line

- Pediatric succinylcholine-associated bradycardia has few documented clinically significant effects and indiscriminate atropine pre-medication provides little clinical benefit.
- Atropine in the setting of repeated doses of a paralyzing agent may decrease the risk of associated bradycardias.
- Optimizing intubating conditions and assuring adequate preoxygenation will mitigate prolonged bradycardia events associated with hypoxia.
- Atropine is associated with ventricular arrhythmias and malignant hyperthermia in infants.

Shellfish allergies contraindicate administration of iodinated contrast

Jennifer Lee, Ryan Pedigo

The Origin

The supposed correlation between shellfish allergies and contrast reactions stems from the commonly held belief of cross-reactivity between iodinated intravenous contrast used for radiographic studies and other substances rich in iodine. Since shellfish provides a rich source of dietary iodine, allergic reactions to contrast became logically linked with the common shellfish allergy.

The basis of this myth, although difficult to trace, most likely originates from a prospective study in 1975 by Shehadi looking at IV contrast reactions. This study highlighted the finding that patients with history of contrast reactions also reported a history of seafood allergies. However, within the study they also reported similar rates of other food allergens.[164]

Many patients with shellfish allergies describe a reaction to IV contrast administration that mirrors reactions they experience after eating shellfish. Thus, many conclude that an "iodine allergy" must be the culprit. Healthcare professionals further propagate the myth by screening for history of shellfish allergies prior to the administration of contrast.[165]

The Facts

Although shellfish contains high concentrations of iodine, it is highly unlikely that the iodine causes any associated hypersensitivity reactions.[166] After all, iodine is naturally present throughout the body within thyroid hormones and iodine is essential for life. Immunologic studies have shown that tropomyosins, found within the muscle cells of shellfish, not iodine, mediate the allergic reaction. There has been no evidence to suggest that these compounds are related to any compounds in iodinated contrast. Furthermore, iodine is an element without three-dimensional molecular structure capable of promoting production of antibodies to facilitate an allergic reaction.[165]

That is not to say that patients with a seafood allergy are at zero risk for a contrast reaction. Patients with unrelated food or environmental allergies, even with no known reaction to prior contrast media administration, may experience a greater risk of developing an allergic reaction to contrast.[167] Regardless of other food or environmental hypersensitivity reactions, and due to the rarity of contrast allergies in general, the American College of Radiology does not recommended withholding contrast studies pre-medicating patients with unrelated allergies.[167] Also the increasingly common use of low-osmolality contrast agents has decreased severe adverse reactions to contrast.[168,169]

The Bottom Line

- No evidence suggests a significant relationship between shellfish allergy and an IV contrast allergy.

- Contrast studies should not be withheld due to a reported shellfish or iodine allergy.
- There is no need to screen for shellfish allergies before administration of IV contrast.

Tamsulosin should be prescribed to all patients with ureteral stones

James H. Williams, Ryan Pedigo

The Origin

Ureteral colic is a common and painful condition seen in the emergency department, and medical expulsion therapy (MET) with alpha-blockers such as tamsulosin has been used for aiding in the passage of ureteral stones for several years. The American Urologic Association and European Association of Urology both currently recommend the use of MET with alpha-blockers to facilitate the passage of ureteral stones.[170,171] The American Urologic Association's 2016 recommendation concludes with a grade B recommendation that tamsulosin be used to facilitate in the passage of any distal ureteral stone <10 mm.[170] Despite the frequent use of tamsulosin for ureteral colic, there remains substantial debate regarding the efficacy of MET for ureteral stones.

The Facts

Early evidence supporting the use of tamsulosin for MET stems from several meta-analyses that showed an apparent benefit for alpha-blockers in passage of ureteral stones. However, many of the studies included in these meta-analyses were small, prone to biases including lack of blinding and incomplete data, and there was substantial heterogeneity of the included studies.[170,172–175] Recently, several more well-designed randomized controlled trials (RCTs) have demonstrated no apparent benefit for tamsulosin with regards to stone passage.[176–178] However, some evidence suggests that a subset of patients with larger stones may benefit from tamsulosin therapy.

A recent meta-analysis of 8 high-quality double-blind, placebo-controlled RCTs found a benefit to MET among patients with stones larger than 5 mm.[179] Similarly, the largest RCT to date, which included 3450 individuals, found a benefit for tamsulosin for individuals with stones larger than 5 mm but no benefit for stones smaller than 5 mm.[180] The high rate of spontaneous passage of small ureteral stones likely accounts for the lack of apparent benefit seen with tamsulosin when used to aid small stone passage. The majority of studies have focused primarily on stone passage as the primary outcome, but several studies examined pain relief as a secondary outcome and identified a possible benefit,[180,181] while others found no benefit. [177,178,182,183] There may be a benefit in the subgroup of larger stones which was diluted by the high prevalence of smaller stones, which did not show benefit. Based on the best available evidence in 2019, tamsulosin can be considered for large (>5mm) and distal ureteral stones (e.g. close to the bladder).

Side-effects of tamsulosin occur at a rate of 6.6%, and include dizziness, hypotension, and retrograde ejaculation.[184] Therefore, prescribing tamsulosin in groups that are not known to benefit exposes them to potential harms without increasing expulsion rates.

The Bottom Line

- Urological professional societies currently recommend the use of tamsulosin for distal ureteral stones <10 mm.
- Administration of MET has significant adverse effects.
- The highest quality RCTs demonstrate a possible increased expulsion rate with medical therapy for patients with stones larger than 5 mm or distal ureteral stones.
- Small stones are likely to pass spontaneously regardless of MET.

Epinephrine cannot be used for digital or penile local anesthesia

Alexander Garrett, Ryan Pedigo

The Origin

Local anesthetics in combination with epinephrine can provide enhanced anesthesia due to local vasoconstriction through alpha-1 receptor stimulation. This increases the duration of anesthetic effect by lowering the rate of local anesthetic clearance, and provides a chemical tourniquet effect, enhancing the efficacy of local nerve blocks.[185,186] A commonly taught axiom is to avoid the use of epinephrine-containing agents in areas of the body served by terminal vessels, (e.g. the "fingers, nose, penis, toes" axiom) due to concerns of inducing tissue ischemia and possibly necrosis. This teaching was formalized in a prominent textbook of hand surgery in 1956, which stated that the use of epinephrine in the digits was contraindicated.[187] Adding to the fear of epinephrine, 50 cases published between 1889 and 1948 described cases of digit necrosis and gangrene following digit blocks.[188–192]

The Facts

The American Academy of Dermatology recommends the use of epinephrine with local anesthetic for use on the ears, nose, hands, feet, and digits. Further, they recommend the consideration of these mixtures for use in penile blocks. They base this recommendation on years of retrospective studies, prospective randomized controlled trials, and literature reviews evaluating the safety of epinephrine's use in the hand and digits.[192,193] One review explains that the original case reports of ischemia with digit blocks were produced in an era wrought with confounding factors, such as prolonged tourniquet use, the practice of dipping injured fingers in boiling water, and the practice of self-mixing epinephrine and anesthetic agents.[192] In least 2797 reported cases of epinephrine's use for digital block since 1958, *no complications have occurred.*

Furthermore, several publications have examined the rate of tissue ischemia and necrosis reported with accidental discharge into a digit of 1:1000 epinephrine auto-injections.[194,195] A 59-patient case series found no associated digital necrosis.[195] If a solution of epinephrine 100x the concentration used for anesthesia (1:100,000) caused no lasting sequelae then the use of doses orders of magnitude lower can be presumed safe. Although most likely unnecessary, phentolamine, an alpha-adrenergic antagonist, can provide pharmacologic rescue by reversing epinephrine induced vasoconstriction.[195–198]

Most studies examining the effects of epinephrine-containing anesthetic agents in patients with baseline vasculopathy also note minimal to no adverse events. A retrospective review of 6 patients examined the use of epinephrine for digital blocks in a population which included many with vasculopathies, and reported no digital ischemia or necrosis.[199] Although far from randomized, a prospective trial focusing on safety in vasculopathic patients concluded that gross harm from epinephrine is unlikely. Further, despite expert endorsement of epinephrine for penile nerve blocks,[185] only one published study examined the safety of this practice, with no observed lasting ischemic complications.[200]

The Bottom Line

- Use of epinephrine-containing local anesthetic agents for digital nerve blocks does not cause acute tissue necrosis or ischemia.
- For patients with vascular disease, additional care should be taken, although epinephrine-induced ischemia is unlikely.
- Although likely unnecessary, subcutaneous infiltration of phentolamine can be used to shorten the duration of vasoconstriction.
- Epinephrine-containing anesthetics most likely do not induce acute penile ischemia due to the high degree of vascularity.

Ketorolac IV/IM provides more effective analgesia than oral NSAIDs

Omid Adibnazari, Ryan Pedigo

The Origin

Ketorolac, a nonsteroidal anti-inflammatory drug (NSAID), w
developed in 1989 and was approved for medical use in the U.S
the same year. Although several parenteral NSAIDs were
available outside of the U.S., ketorolac was the first FDA-
approved parenteral NSAID. Numerous studies have
demonstrated its analgesic potency on the level of a low-dose
opioid, with exceptional efficacy in renal colic,[201,202] blunt
extremity trauma,[203] and for postoperative setting pain.[204–206]
Additionally, many healthcare providers believe that patients
perceive intravenous/intramuscular (IV/IM) medications to be
stronger than oral medications, and that this perception results
improved analgesia. Consequently, parenteral ketorolac has
become a widely used analgesic in emergency departments an
frequently chosen over oral NSAIDs.

The Facts

Parenteral ketorolac and oral ibuprofen have similar efficacy
for analgesia. Both medications work by the same mechanism,
sharing nearly identical pharmacodynamics and very similar
pharmacokinetics regardless of administration route. While one
the earliest comparison studies in 1994 demonstrated greater
analgesia with ketorolac after strabismus surgery, the methods

had notable flaws.[207] Significant shortcomings included different timing of doses, as well as alteration of the commercially available form of ibuprofen, which may have interfered with its normal pharmacodynamics. The same year, an emergency-department-based study evaluating patients with acute pain from a variety of complaints demonstrated near identical efficacy of 800 mg of oral ibuprofen and 60 mg of IM ketorolac.[208] A double-blind, randomized trial the following year showed equivalent analgesia with 800 mg of oral ibuprofen and 60 mg of IV ketorolac in ED patients with acute traumatic musculoskeletal pain.[209] Another ED study in 1998 showed similar results, with no difference in pain levels between the two medications.[210] Several studies have shown no difference in pain control in postoperative patients using IV/IM ketorolac or oral ibuprofen.[211,212]

Providers often administer parenteral ketorolac instead of oral NSAIDs to gain an additional placebo effect from the perception that an injection must provide greater pain relief. One interesting randomized, double-blind study investigated this phenomenon by providing trauma patients oral or IM placebo. All patients also received oral ibuprofen dissolved in a flavored beverage.[213] They found no significant difference in pain reduction when patients thought they were getting an IM analgesic. Ketorolac, therefore, should not be given solely for the perceived benefit of an injection when oral alternatives suffice.

Ketorolac also carries the greatest gastrointestinal bleeding risk of all the NSAIDS, especially in patients older than 60 years of age.[214–216] This risk may be mitigated using lower but equally efficacious doses. The traditionally high 30mg or 60mg doses of ketorolac greatly exceed the pharmacologic ceiling for effective analgesia. In 2017, a randomized double-blind trial demonstrated a therapeutic ceiling of 10mg for ketorolac, obviating the need to consider potentially harmful higher doses.[217]

The Bottom Line

- Ketorolac provides excellent analgesia, and for many conditions has an efficacy equivalent to low-dose opioid medications.
- Oral ibuprofen provides equivalent analgesia to IM/IV ketorolac
- Ketorolac use carries a greater risk of gastrointestinal bleeding than other NSAIDs.
- There is unlikely to be any additional placebo benefit from giving IV or IM NSAIDs compared to an oral NSAID.

Patients with stable angina benefit from PCI

Alexander S. Grohmann, Ryan Pedigo

The Origin

Percutaneous cardiac intervention (PCI) has remained the cornerstone for the treatment of coronary artery disease and myocardial infarction (MI) in conjunction with medication. PCI has great success in decreasing mortality of patients with ST-segment elevation MI by stenting the culprit coronary lesion. In addition, there appears to be benefit in primary PCI for significant non-culprit lesions found during intervention for STEMI.[218] This led to the reasonable assumption that stenting lesions of patients with stable angina would also provide a benefit. Opening a significantly obstructed coronary artery could theoretically provide a higher quality of life with decreased anginal symptoms, reduced risk of myocardial infarction, and improved cardiac function.

The Facts

PCI for stable angina, unfortunately, has not been shown to reduce the incidence of MI, mortality, or daily symptoms in patients compared to optimized medical therapy (OMT). OMT consists of daily aspirin, a beta-blocker, an ACE inhibitor, and possibly an additional antiplatelet therapy if post-PCI. Although multiple studies had suggested this conclusion, the first large meta-analysis published in 2005 pooled data from 11 smaller studies and concluded that, in patients with stable angina on OMT, PCI did not decrease the risk of death, MI or need for future revascularization.[219] The landmark COURAGE trial randomized 2287 patients to PCI or OMT over a 4.6-year period and evaluated for the primary end point of death and rate of nonfatal MI. This study also found that PCI for stable angina offered no decrease in death or MI when compared to OMT.[220]

The FAME-2 randomized trial challenged this consensus, suggesting that certain patients with stable angina may benefit from PCI: in patients with stable angina on OMT with fractional flow reserve (degree of blood flow through a stenotic coronary artery) ≤0.80, PCI reduced the rate of death, nonfatal MI and need for urgent revascularization.[221] However, the composite outcome was largely met by the need for urgent revascularization, primarily performed due to symptoms. This trial demonstrates the danger of composite outcomes. Death, nonfatal MI, and urgent revascularization all meet the composite outcome but are not truly equally important (e.g., death is worse than needing urgent revascularization).

While PCI for stable angina does not reduce risk of MI, risk of death, or admissions for acute coronary syndromes, questions have arisen whether PCI may improve quality of life by decreasing angina symptoms. The COURAGE research included assessment of quality of life in patients who were randomized to either PCI or OMT for stable angina. The patients randomized to PCI demonstrated a period of decreased angina during the first 24 months of intervention. At 36 months the patients in the PCI arm experienced no less angina than those on OMT.[222]

To help further clarify the effects of PCI on angina, the ORBITA trial, a multicenter double-blind randomized trial of 200 patients compared angiography-guided PCI versus angiography without PCI (sham PCI). Patients were evaluated before and after intervention objectively with treadmill exercise time testing and subjectively with perception of impact on quality of life. There were no significant differences between groups in both objective and subjective measures at 6 weeks post-intervention.[223] Of note, the study has drawn criticism since the patients had less severe disease compared to prior studies, the sample size was small, the follow up period was short, and the interval check-in of three times a week does not represent typical medical practice—all these factors may have influenced patients' perception of symptoms. Despite the controversy, the conclusions are similar to those in the COURAGE trial—PCI offers no benefit to patients with stable angina when compared to medical therapy.

The Bottom Line

- PCI for patients with stable angina does not decrease mortality from cardiovascular events.
- Optimization of medical therapy without PCI is the appropriate course of action for the initial treatment of patients with stable coronary artery disease.
- PCI may be beneficial in patients with fractional flow reserve of ≤0.80 on optimal medical therapy.

Orthostatic vital signs predict hypovolemia

Jackie Shibata, Ryan Pedigo

The Origin

When a person stands up, approximately 300-800 mL of blood pools in the lower extremities, resulting in decreased venous return, stroke volume and cardiac output. The body responds through neurovascular mechanisms by increasing sympathetic response and decreasing vagal tone in an attempt to maintain cardiac output.[224] During states of extreme volume depletion, patients may have decreased cardiac output upon standing as a result of the larger-than-expected decrease in preload.[225] Thus, hypovolemic person may be expected to develop orthostatic hypotension.

Orthostatic hypotension (OH) was originally defined as a sign of hypovolemia, of which patients may or may not have symptoms. Formally, OH occurs when systolic blood pressure (SBP) declines by ≥20mmHg or a diastolic blood pressure (DBP) by ≥10mmHg within 3 minutes of standing or a head-up tilt greater than 60°.[226] This definition was produced by expert consensus and was intended for use in the diagnosis of neurogenic orthostatic hypotension: postural drops in blood pressure as a result of inadequate release of catecholamines or vasoconstrictor failure.[224] These experts note that many other variables such as diurnal patterns, food ingestion, age, medications, ambient temperature, gender, prolonged recumbence and deconditioning affect postural vital signs.[224]

Despite these confounders and lack of gold-standard comparisons, this consensus-developed measurement was adopted for evaluation of volume status and is still recommended by emergency medicine textbooks and cardiology association guidelines.[227–230]

The Facts

Since the 1980s, observational studies have shown an association between OH and volume depletion.[231–233] However, OH is not just associated with hypovolemia. In normal, healthy, non-hypovolemic volunteers, orthostatic hypotension can occur. Ooi et al. found >50% of non-hospitalized nursing home residents (n = 911) met criteria for OH.[234] Another study found 44% of healthy adolescent volunteers, with normal vasoconstrictive function, had positive OH during a head-up tilt table test at 70°.[230] Therefore, the presence of OH does not always signify hypovolemia.

The lack of OH has a similarly poor negative predictive value for volume depletion. One study found that only 17% of healthy blood donors met criteria for OH after a 10% intravascular volume loss (450 mL blood donation).[235] A systematic review evaluating the operating characteristics of orthostatic hypotension in phlebotomized patients who lost 450 to 630 mL of blood concluded OH had a sensitivity of 9% (95%CI 6-12) in younger subjects and 27% (95%CI 14-40) in subjects >65 years old. The positive (LR+) and negative (LR-) likelihood ratios for OH were LR+ 1.8 and LR- 1.0 in younger subjects and LR+ 1.9 and LR-

0.9 in older subjects.[236] These findings suggest post-test probabilities for hypovolemia are essentially unchanged after measuring orthostatic vital signs. Therefore, there is no utility in performing this exam when evaluating for hypovolemia.

Despite this evidence, the 2017 ACC/AHA/HRS Guideline for the Evaluation and Management of Patients with Syncope recommends checking orthostatic vital signs on all patients presenting with syncope.[227] For those found to have OH related to neurogenic OH or hypovolemic causes, rehydration treatment is recommended (Class I evidence). However, these guidelines fail to include the level of evidence or any supporting literature for the recommendation to use OH to primarily diagnose these conditions from the outset. Additionally, Bloom et al. assert these guidelines offer no evidence that positive OH testing can discriminate between life-threatening and low-risk causes of syncope.[237] Since some patients will have OH at baseline, this may lead to inappropriate early diagnostic closure.

In summary, OH testing has a long history and sound theoretical and physiologic basis, which has resulted in continued recommendation for use in both medical textbooks and practice guidelines. However, this sign was developed from consensus opinion informed by small observational studies from the 1990s and has never been formally tested against a gold standard or for evaluation of patient outcomes or patient's perception of presyncope attributable to hypovolemia.[229] The presence or absence of OH cannot accurately diagnose or exclude hypovolemia.

The Bottom Line

- Orthostatic hypotension is based on expert opinion and has not been tested against a gold standard.
- Many variables including neurologic dysfunction cause orthostatic hypotension and euvolemic patients may also manifest with the finding.
- Orthostatic vital sign testing has a very poor predictive value for diagnosing hypovolemia and it is frequently absent in patients with significant volume loss.

Ceftriaxone IM for gonorrhea has a depot effect

Daniel G. Ostermayer

The Origin

The Centers for Disease Control and Prevention (CDC) recommends intramuscular (IM) ceftriaxone as the preferred treatment for acute *N. gonorrhoeae* infections. This recommendation has led many clinicians to assume that the IM application is as important as the 250 mg dosing because of a sustained release (depot effect) from the IM injection. Patients who may have an intravenous catheter for other reasons (such a lab draw) and also require treatment for gonorrhea, often receive an IM injection despite having an established IV route.

The Facts

Gonorrhea historically (1930s) was susceptible to sulfonamides. Initial limitations on effectiveness were followed b a decline. Penicillin became the preferred treatment in the '40s, until resistance appeared in the '60s, attributed (1976) to the bacteria's production of beta-lactamase and independently (198 to genetic mutation. Afterwards, tetracyclines were effective unt resistance developed, when fluroquinolones were used.[238] In th 2000s, fluoroquinolones also became ineffective. The CDC first recommended against fluoroquinolone use in Asia and the Pac Islands, and then in 2004 throughout the United States. At that time, cephalosporins became the most effective and widely available therapy. Oral cephalosporins such as cefixime had a short window of efficacy before gonorrhea rapidly developed resistance.[239] In 2010, the CDC recommended increasing the once-effective dose of ceftriaxone 125 mg IM to 250 mg IM.[240] Ultimately, treatment of gonorrhea requires exceeding the minimal inhibitory concentration (MIC) in addition to duration of exposure.[241] According to the CDC, ceftriaxone has an MIC for *N. gonorrhoeae* of 0.125 μg/mL. Since 2006, resistant strains of *N. gonorrhoeae* with MICs $\geq$ 0.125 μg/ml, although still rare, have been detected and may require further increases in ceftriaxone dosing or even complete abandonment of cephalosporins.[242] Per the U.S. Food and Drug Administration, both IV and IM ceftriaxone at 500 mg doses exceed the MICs set forth by the CDC for both newly evolved and more common sensitive strains.

Ceftriaxone plasma concentrations after a single dose (µg/mL)							
Dose & Route	0.5 hr	1hr	2hr	4hr	8hr	12hr	24
0.5 gm IV	82	59	48	37	23	15	24
0.5 gm IM (250mg/ml)	22	33	38	35	26	16	5
0.5 gm IM (350 mg/mL)	20	32	38	34	24	16	5

A third to two thirds of ceftriaxone is excreted in the urine as bioactive drug. Both the IV and IM routes also exceed the required bactericidal MICs in the urine.[243]

Ceftriaxone plasma concentrations after a single dose (µg/mL)					
Dose & Route	0-2 hr	2-4 hr	8-12 hr	12-24 hr	24-48h
0.5 gm IV	526	366	87	70	15
0.5 gm IM	115	425	127	96	28

In patients with renal insufficiency, the plasma concentration will remain higher than patients with normal glomerular filtration rates regardless of IV or IM routes.[244] Although the plasma concentrations of a 250 mg IV dose of ceftriaxone are not published, it is at least as effective to treat gonorrhea patients with 500 mg of IV ceftriaxone.

The Bottom Line
- Ceftriaxone 500 mg IV exceeds the MIC required to treat *N. gonorrhoeae*

- The recommendation for IM ceftriaxone originates from the growing resistance of gonorrhea, not from an intramuscular depot effect.

Patients with acute intracranial hemorrhage benefit from immediate blood pressure reduction

Manpreet Singh, Daniel Ostermayer

The Origin

The human body's reaction to acute intracranial hemorrhage was originally described over a century ago by Harvey Cushing. Acute intracranial blood induces an often rapid increa in arterial systolic blood pressure.[245] Since prognosis for acute non traumatic intracranial hemorrhage (ICH) depends on the location and size of the bleed, emergency department management has focused partly on therapies that might limit hemorrhage size and expansion. Although an acute hypertensi response occurs in response to ICH, blood pressure reduction was originally proposed as a means of limiting hematoma volur and reducing mortality. The American Stroke Association in 199 suggested emergent blood pressure control in patients with acu ICH based largely on expert opinion.[246] This practice of aggressive blood pressure control during ICH, gained even greater adoption after publication of the pilot INTERACT-1 trial and incorporation into American Heart Association (AHA) guidelines.[248] INTERACT-1 randomized patients to receive targ systolic blood pressures of 180 mmHg or 140 mmHg. The study was not powered to detect a clinical outcome but was rather focused on feasibility. The study found a statistically non-significant difference of 1.7 mL in ICH volume between the groups.

The original scientific basis for the safety of reducing blood pressure despite the body's hypertensive response to ICH predates INTERACT-1. Animal data and neuroimaging studies suggested that, although tissues experience hypoperfusion from ICH, there is not an ischemic penumbra surrounding the hemorrhage.[249] Therefore, if blood pressure reduction could decrease the expansion of intracranial hemorrhage, it would do so without causing further damage to surrounding tissue (since there is no ischemic penumbra at risk of hypoperfusion).

The Facts

The best available data regarding the safety and efficacy of acute blood pressure lowering in ICH originates from two randomized double-blind trials: INTERACT-2 and ATACH-2. Of important note, across these trials patients with structural causes of ICH such as arteriovenous malformations, intracranial aneurysms, and masses were excluded. Following promising results from INTERACT-1, in terms of reducing hematoma size,[247] researchers developed INTERACT-2.[250] This study randomized 2839 patients who presented within 6 hours of spontaneous ICH with elevated systolic blood pressure (SBP) to either standard treatment (target systolic <180 mmHg) or intensive treatment (target systolic <140 mmHg) within one hour of diagnosis and for a duration of 7 days. There were no major differences in adverse effects, namely mortality or neurologic deterioration, between the two groups.

This study was largely presented by the authors as positive, supporting the safety of intensive blood pressure lowering. However, it did now show any patient-centered benefits. There were no statistically significant differences between the two groups in their primary endpoint, death or disability (defined by modified Rankin score) at 90 days. Additionally, no difference i hematoma size was found in the subgroup that underwent repe CT scanning at 24 hours. The INTERACT-2 authors did howev find a trend toward lower modified Rankin scores in the intensiv treatment group. This was only found after an ordinal analysis was performed, a statistical method that assumes knowledge c patient baseline, which was unknown for most if not all enrollec patients.[251–253]

Then, the ATACH-2 trial confirmed the null results of INTERACT-2. In ATACH-2, 1,000 patients with intracranial hemorrhage, a GCS $\geq$5, and presenting within 4.5 hours with hypertension (SBP > 180 mmHg) were randomized to standarc treatment (SBP 140-179 mmHg) or intensive lowering (SBP 11 139 mmHg) using nicardipine as the first-line medication.[254] Of note, the trial also excluded patients with severe hypertension (defined as SBP > 240 mmHg on two readings) and those with ICH of unknown onset. The study found no statistically significa difference between the two groups for its primary outcome of death and disability (modified Rankin score 4-6) at 90 days an was stopped early due to futility. There were also no statistically significant differences in secondary outcomes of hematoma expansion or neurologic deterioration within 24 hours. Patients in the intensive treatment arm experienced greater incidence of acute kidney injury (9% vs 4%).[254]

By all measures, ATACH-2 was a much more robust clinical trial than INTERACT-2. All participants in ATACH-2 were randomized earlier after onset of symptoms (all within 4.5 hours vs 41% within 4 hours in INTERACT-2), all had initial SBP > 180 mmHg (vs only 48% in INTERACT-2). ATACH-2 also had fewer treatment failures. It is important to note, however, that these results cannot be generalized to patients with severe hypertension (SBP > 240 mmHg), aneurysmal related bleeding, intraventricular hemorrhage, GCS <5, and traumatic ICH. Although acute blood pressure lowering in the setting of ICH is safe, no robust trial has ever demonstrated any patient-centered benefit.

The Bottom Line

- Aggressive reduction of systolic blood pressure to 140 mmHg offers no clinical benefit over guideline targets of 180 mmHg for spontaneous, non-traumatic, non-structural-lesion-induced ICH.
- The guideline-suggested blood pressure target of 180 mmHg for ICH originates from expert consensus and physiologic reasoning.

- Acute blood pressure reduction to the goal of <180 mmHg ma[y]
  decrease hematoma expansion but without obvious patient-
  centered benefits.
- Blood pressure control for ICH does appear relatively safe
  regardless of clinical efficacy.

Chronic alcoholics require a banana bag

Huy A. Phan, Jonathan Giordano

The Origin

Patients with chronic alcohol abuse or the acutely intoxicated often receive an IV banana bag during their ED stay to correct presumed vitamin deficiencies.[255,256] The banana bag traditionally contains 1 L solution of 5% dextrose, saline, 100 mg of thiamine, 1 mg of folic acid, 2 gm of magnesium sulfate, and a dissolved multivitamin tablet. The B-vitamins provide the characteristic yellow color resulting in the bag's common name. The banana bag was historically used in the treatment of vitamin and electrolyte deficiencies in patients with terminal illnesses and in chronic alcoholics admitted to the intensive care unit.

The Facts

The use of the banana bag in chronic alcoholics presenting to the emergency department, although a longstanding and common practice, carries a high cost with no therapeutic benefit. Alcohol abusers can develop vitamin deficiencies due to poor diet, underlying liver disease, and alcohol's effects on intestinal absorption of nutrients. These deficiencies, although rare, can include folate and/or vitamin B_{12} deficiencies causing megaloblastic anemia or thiamine deficiency leading to Wernicke-Korsakoff Syndrome (WKS). A prospective, observational study at Jacobi Medical Center reveals that no patients with acute alcohol intoxication had a folate or a vitamin B_{12} deficiency.[257]

Also, the banana bag only contains 100 mg of thiamine, a dose insufficient in preventing Wernicke-Korsakoff Syndrome.[256,258] Treatment of WKS requires 200–500 mg IV thiamine every 8 hours.

The consequences of these vitamin deficiencies develop over time, and rarely correct acutely with IV supplementation. The bioavailability of oral folic acid and multivitamins approach 100% with a dramatically lower cost than IV formulations. Thiamine, however, due to deficiencies in intestinal absorption in alcoholic requires IV administration for maximal effectiveness.[255,259] The banana bag is also supplemented with magnesium, another deficiency that alcoholics frequently develop. There is little evidence that prophylactic magnesium supplementation offers clinical benefits unless severe deficiency is confirmed by laboratory testing or associated with concomitant hypokalemia.[255,256,260]

Providers also may also assume that the banana bag provide the IV fluids necessary to expedite sobriety. A randomized controlled trial on 144 emergency department patients found no difference in length of stay, treatment time, change of breath alcohol level, or intoxication score in patients who received IV fluids compared to patients who were simply observed.[261] Regardless of administration of fluids, the body metabolizes alcohol at a fixed hourly rate governed by zero order kinetics.[262]

The Bottom Line

- The 100 mg of IV thiamine in a banana bag insufficiently treats or prevents Wernicke-Korsakoff syndrome.
- Folic acid and multivitamins have similar bioavailability regardless of route.
- The banana bag offers no clinical benefits and exposes the patient to unnecessary interventions at high cost.

Health insurance will not pay the bill if a patient leaves AMA

Daniel G. Ostermayer

The Origin

Many U.S. healthcare providers and patients alike worry that their health insurance will not cover the hospital bill if they leave against medical advice (AMA). Occasionally the threat of having an unpaid bill is used to dissuade a patient from leaving prior to completion of their workup. This belief extends to inpatient ward as well as the emergency department. At the University of Chicago, 43.9% of surveyed attendings and 68.6% of residents believed that if a patient left the inpatient service AMA, insuranc would not pay the bill. Providers stated that they learned about his myth from a multitude of sources including case managers, other residents and attendings.[263]

The Facts

Two studies provide evidence that, regardless of public or private insurance, leaving AMA from a hospital does not incur a refusal of payment. In a letter to the editor in 2008, a suburban level I trauma center performed a retrospective review of 104 consecutive cases of patients with insurance leaving against medical advice. Patients' insurance spanned 19 different companies and included HMOs, PPOs, Medicare, and Medicaid All were reimbursed.[264]

For inpatients, the results were similar. During the Hospitalists Study (comparing costs when patients received treatment from traditional internists vs hospitalists) at the University of Chicago[265] 1% of the 46,319 patients left AMA. Of the AMA patients, 4% had insurance deny their claim, but not because they left AMA. Often the payment refusal occurred due to an administrative mistake such as wrong name or insurance information. Although it is possible that the insurance company did not truthfully cite the reason for denial and instead claimed administrative issues, this seemed unlikely since the majority of the 18 patients with denied payment had non-private (Medicare/Medicaid) insurance.[265]

The Bottom Line

- Health insurance companies in the U.S. do not deny coverage if a patient leaves the hospital AMA.

Ketamine raises intracranial pressure and should be avoided in patients with traumatic brain injury

Daniel G. Ostermayer

The Origin

Ketamine, as both an induction agent and procedural sedative has historically been avoided in patients with or at risk of traumatic brain injury (TBI) due to the fear of increasing intracranial pressure (ICP). During intracranial hemorrhage or cerebral contusion, the tissue surrounding the insult is at increased risk for injury due to disruption in blood flow autoregulation. Therefore, large increases in cerebral perfusion pressure (CPP) could further exacerbate a traumatic brain injury by increasing intracranial pressure.[266,267]

In 1971, Gardner et al. describes 11 surgeries in healthy male who received 2 mg/kg ketamine-facilitated anesthesia for orthopedic or hemorrhoid-related procedures. The ICP was measured via intraoperative lumbar pressure transducers and the study reported a mean increase in 18 mmHg and a mean arterial pressure increase of 28 mmHg. In 1972, a second publication described 20 patients with ICP pressure measurements during lumbar discectomy facilitated by ketamine (1.1 mg/kg) and nitro oxide general anesthesia. In 6 of the 9 patients with space-occupying brain lesions, increases in ICP occurred (increase in 12 mmHg).[268] Multiple other case series during the 1970s describe patients with intracranial pathologies such as hydrocephalus or intracranial masses who experienced ICP increases when provided with similar 1–2 mg/kg of ketamine during operative procedures.[269–272]

The Facts

Since the original case reports and series, multiple randomized trials have examined the use of ketamine sedation in patients with traumatic brain injuries and mass lesions. Although none of the studies were performed in patients undergoing rapid sequence intubation (RSI), and all include the use of a second analgesic or sedative, none show statistical increases in ICP or CPP pressure during the administration of ketamine.

Bourgain et al. conducted two randomized controlled trials (RCTs) providing the best evidence that ketamine with midazolam as a continuous infusion does not elevate ICP or provide any significant increase in CPP.[273,274] The first, a study published in 2003, compared patients with TBI requiring mechanical ventilation and ICP monitoring with GCS < 9. Patients were randomized to sedation with ketamine and midazolam or sufentanil and midazolam infusions. No significant difference was found in mean daily ICP or CPP between groups.[274] Similarly, in a second trial using target controlled infusions to measure plasma sedative levels, patients with GCS <9 and TBI were randomized to sufentanil-midazolam or ketamine-midazolam infusions. No differences in the mean ICP or CPP occurred between groups.[273]

One RCT comparing ketamine-midazolam infusions vs fentanyl-midazolam infusions in patients with TBI found a 2 mmHg ICP increase (8 mm Hg increase in CPP) in the ketamine group. The clinical significance of this effect was not reported.[27] In patients sedated with propofol, bolus doses of ketamine did n increase ICP or CPP.[276] Similarly, neurosurgical patients undergoing craniotomy for intracranial masses given bolus dose (1 mg/kg) of ketamine did not experience ICP or CPP increases.[277] Although no RCT has evaluated ICP changes during RSI, the potential blood pressure elevations caused by ketamine could protect against especially harmful hypotensive events during intubation.[278]

The Bottom Line

- Early case reports of ketamine-induced ICP and CPP elevation have not been replicated with more modern RCTs.
- Ketamine infusions paired with a benzodiazepine do not eleva ICP or CPP.
- Ketamine bolus dosing during sedation also does not elevate ICP or CPP.

Corticosteroids treat anaphylaxis and prevent biphasic reactions

Kerollos A. Shaker, Jonathan Giordano, Daniel G. Ostermayer

The Origin

Anaphylactic reactions after the initial mast cell degranulation phase may have a secondary event (biphasic reaction) occur within 72 hours. This reaction can occur without re-exposure to the originating trigger, is generally reported with an incidence of 3-23%, and often occurs within 6–11 hours.[279] Historically, administration of steroids, specifically glucocorticoids, was thought to prevent occurrence of the biphasic event via a multitude of physiologic pathways in addition to decreasing anaphylactic severity. This included downregulation of IgE expression and decreased mast cell activation, the key components in anaphylaxis.[280] From a physiologic standpoint, since corticosteroids downregulate the inflammatory response and have a longer duration of action than epinephrine, they could reduce the severity of the initial event and inhibit development of a biphasic reaction. This has led to often routine administration of glucocorticoids (methylprednisolone, prednisone, or dexamethasone) in addition to epinephrine to treat anaphylaxis.

The Facts

To date, no randomized clinical trial has tested the assumption that steroids provide benefit during the acute phase or for a biphasic reaction.[281,282] Prednisone, dexamethasone, and methylprednisolone have a delayed effect with bioavailability occurring within 1-2 hours after administration,[283,284] thus limiting their usefulness during the acute phase and potentially delaying the administration of epinephrine. The American Academy of Allergy, Asthma and Immunology (AAAAI) states that corticosteroids have no role in the acute management of anaphylaxis.[285]

Patients at greatest risk for a subsequent biphasic reaction are those who have an unknown trigger or presented to the ED with hypotension.[286] Underdosing and delayed dosing of epinephrine combined with initial severity of anaphylaxis reaction most likely *increase* the risk of occurrence of a biphasic reaction in both adults and children.[287] Early, especially prehospital, epinephrine administration can substantially decrease the duration of anaphylaxis and may be the most effective therapy at decreasing the risk of a biphasic reaction.[288–291]

Regarding prevention of biphasic reactions, again, no randomized trials have evaluated effectiveness, but a review of 21 studies of lesser quality found no decrease in biphasic reaction incidence or duration with glucocorticoid administration. One prospective ED-based study evaluated 134 patients with a diagnosis of allergic reaction or anaphylaxis with respect to biphasic reactions and steroid administration. Overall 19.4% experienced a biphasic reaction, with a median time to occurrence of 10 hours. Although not statistically significant, one

35% of the group with a biphasic reaction received steroids vs 55% with a uniphasic event. However, the biphasic group also received less epinephrine.

Some concern exists with respect to pediatric patients having a greater risk of biphasic reactions than adults, but a review of 5,203 cases found no significant difference in return ED visits within 72 hours between those who received steroids compared to those without administration.[292] Also, multiple studies have failed to find a difference in steroid route or formulation with respect to decreasing the occurrence of biphasic reactions.[293–297]

Despite lack of evidence for and much evidence against effectiveness, many providers may still opt to provide a single dose or short course of steroids due to a perceived lack of harm. Dosing of steroids in singular or short courses carries the risk of hyperglycemia, dyslipidemia, acute psychosis, pancreatitis, and unnecessary additional financial cost.[298]

The Bottom Line

- Glucocorticoid administration does not decrease the severity of an acute anaphylactic reaction.
- Biphasic reactions are associated with more severe anaphylactic reactions and delayed epinephrine administration.
- Biphasic reactions are not prevented by glucocorticoid administration.

The discriminatory zone predicts success i identifying an IUP

Evan Laveman, Ryan Pedigo

The Origin

The use of transvaginal ultrasound for the evaluation of first trimester symptoms (bleeding, cramping, abdominal pain) reached widespread use in the 1980s. Ultrasound has since become the diagnostic test of choice for determining if a symptomatic patient has a normal IUP, abnormal IUP, or an ectopic pregnancy.[299] Rates of ectopic pregnancy have risen ov the past several decades from 1% of pregnancies, to 2%, due t the increase in the incidence of pelvic inflammatory disease, IUDs, and in vitro fertilization.[300,301] Various proposed beta-hCG discriminatory zones have served as guides for assessing the likelihood of visualizing an IUP on transvaginal ultrasound and have ranged from 1,000-40,000 mIU/mL, with the most quoted being between 1,500-2,000 mIU/mL.[300–302]

In 1994, Barnhart et al, described the 1,500 mIU/mL discriminatory zone after evaluating 1,263 patients. They determined that *all* women with a presenting beta-hCG above 1,500 mIU/mL were accurately diagnosed with an IUP.[303] This diagnostic protocol, however, included outpatient follow up, bet trending, and re-imaging. Although presented as a single diagnostic cutoff, since reevaluations and re-imaging occurred most of the patients, the threshold of 1,500 mIU/mL did not actually serve as a useful diagnostic threshold for a single evaluation. This study could not determine the sensitivity or specificity for making an ultrasound diagnosis on a patient's initial visit.

The Facts

An additional study by Barnhart in 1999 evaluated 333 patients retrospectively, using that same 1,500 mIU/mL beta-hCG threshold.[304] Their data demonstrated that on the initial ultrasound of symptomatic women with beta-hCG levels above 1,500 mIU/mL, a transvaginal ultrasound possessed a specificity of 90.1% (to *rule in* an IUP), and a sensitivity of 80% (to *rule out* an ectopic). This means that after initial evaluation there was a large percentage of women with beta-hCG levels above 1,500 mIU/mL that had a non-diagnostic study. These women either had an early viable IUP, non-viable IUP, or an ectopic pregnancy. The initial 1994 study itself recognized that in its data set, at least 4% of ultimately viable IUPs presenting above the 1,500 mIU/mL threshold were diagnosed on later imaging. Again, this highlights the utility and shortcomings of a threshold of 1,500 mIU/mL.

A 2013 retrospective cohort study with 651 patients at a single site reevaluated the beta-hCG discriminatory zones for patients presenting with first trimester symptoms, and used a logistic regression model to establish beta-hCG cutoffs that would correlate with a 99% probability of visualizing a gestational sac, yolk sac, or fetal pole. These 99% cutoffs were 3,510 (gestational sac), 17,716 (yolk sac), and 47,685 (fetal pole) mIU/mL.[305] A cutoff of 1,500 mIU/mL would have missed 20% of ultimately viable IUPs in their data set and may have resulted in a falsely presumed ectopic. These data lead to the 2018 ACOG recommendation of using a 3,500 mIU/mL as a conservative discriminatory zone.[302]

Although a "discriminatory zone" helps to protocolize the evaluation of a suspected ectopic vs. IUP, the data suggest that no cutoff can perfectly predict the presence of an IUP or absence of an ectopic pregnancy if not visualized with ultrasound. In general, IUP visualization cannot reliably be achieved until beta hCG levels well exceed the previously proposed discriminatory zones of 1,500 mIU/mL.

The Bottom Line

- Recent literature suggests that a beta-hCG threshold of 17-18,000 mIU/mL not the traditional 1,500 mIU/mL would predict >99% likelihood of visualizing a viable IUP with a yolk sac.
- ACOG recommends the use of a beta-hCG discriminatory zone for gestational sac visualization of 3,500 mIU/mL based on 2018 recommendations.
- Given the wide ranges and unreliability of a beta-hCG for predicting IUP visualization, diagnosis or exclusion of an ectopic pregnancy cannot be based on this lab value.

References

1. Herbert ME, Brewster GS, Lanctot-Herbert M. Ten percent of patients who are allergic to penicillin will have serious reactions if exposed to cephalosporins. *West J Med*. 2000;172(5):341.

2. Frumin J, Gallagher JC. Allergic cross-sensitivity between penicillin, carbapenem, and monobactam antibiotics: What are the chances? *Ann Pharmacother*. 2009;43(2):304-315.

3. Goodman EJ, Morgan MJ, Johnson PA, Nichols BA, Denk N, Gold BB. Cephalosporins can be given to penicillin-allergic patients who do not exhibit an anaphylactic response. *J Clin Anesth*. 2001;13(8):561-564.

4. Park MA, Koch CA, Klemawesch P, Joshi A, Li JT. Increased adverse drug reactions to cephalosporins in penicillin allergy patients with positive penicillin skin test. *Int Arch Allergy Immunol*. 2010;153(3):268-273.

5. Miranda A, Blanca M, Vega JM, et al. Cross-reactivity between a penicillin and a cephalosporin with the same side chain. *J Allergy Clin Immunol*. 1996;98(3):671-677.

6. Pichichero ME, Casey JR. Safe use of selected cephalosporins in penicillin-allergic patients: A meta-analysis. *Otolaryngol - Head Neck Surg*. 2007;136(3):340-347.

7. du Plessis T, Walls G, Jordan A, Holland DJ. Implementation of a pharmacist-led penicillin allergy de-labelling service in a public hospital. *J Antimicrob Chemother*. February 2019:1-9.

8. Shenoy ES, Macy E, Rowe T, Blumenthal KG. Evaluation and Management of Penicillin Allergy: A Review. *JAMA*.

2019;321(2):188-199.

9. Niska R, Bhuiya F, Xu J. National hospital ambulatory medical care survey: 2009 emergency department summary. *Natl Hea* *Stat Rep.* 2010;(26):1-31.

10. Singer AJ, Dagum AB. Current Management of Acute Cutaneo' Wounds. *N Engl J Med.* 2008;359(10):1037-1046.

11. Worrall GJ. Repairing skin lacerations: does sterile technique matter? *Can Fam Physician.* 1989;35:790-791.

12. Bodiwala GG, George TK. Surgical Gloves During Wound Repa in the Accident-and-Emergency Department. *Lancet.* 1982;320(8289):91-92.

13. Rutherford WH, Spence RAJ. Infection in wounds sutured in th accident and emergency department. *Ann Emerg Med.* 1980;9(7):350-352.

14. Hollander JE, Singer AJ, Valentine SM, Shofer FS. Risk factors f infection in patients with traumatic lacerations. *Acad Emerg Med.* 2001;8(7):716-720.

15. Perelman VS, Francis GJ, Rutledge T, Foote J, Martino F, Dranitsaris G. Sterile Versus Nonsterile Gloves for Repair of Uncomplicated Lacerations in the Emergency Department: A Randomized Controlled Trial. *Ann Emerg Med.* 2004;43(3):36: 370.

16. Heggers JP, Robson MC, Doran ET. Quantitative assessment o bacterial contamination of open wounds by a slide technique *Trans R Soc Trop Med Hyg.* 1969;63(4):532-534.

17. Creamer J, Davis K, Rice W. Sterile gloves: Do they make a

difference? *Am J Surg*. 2012;204(6):976-980.

18. Gambino SR, Thiede WH. Comparisons of pH in Human Arterial, Venous, and Capillary Blood. *Am J Clin Pathol*. 1959;32(3_ts):298-300.

19. Adrogué HJ, Rashad MN, Gorin AB, Yacoub J, Madias NE. Assessing acid-base status in circulatory failure. Differences between arterial and central venous blood. *N Engl J Med*. 1989;320(20):1312-1316.

20. Weil MH, Rackow EC, Trevino R, Grundler W, Falk JL, Griffel MI. Difference in acid-base state between venous and arterial blood during cardiopulmonary resuscitation. *N Engl J Med*. 1986;315(3):153-156.

21. Mortensen JD. Clinical sequelae from arterial needle puncture, cannulation, and incision. *Circulation*. 1967.

22. McCanny P, Bennett K, Staunton P, McMahon G. Venous vs arterial blood gases in the assessment of patients presenting with an exacerbation of chronic obstructive pulmonary disease. *Am J Emerg Med*. 2012.

23. Zeserson E, Goodgame B, Hess JD, et al. Correlation of Venous Blood Gas and Pulse Oximetry With Arterial Blood Gas in the Undifferentiated Critically Ill Patient. *J Intensive Care Med*. 2016.

24. Kelly AM, McAlpine R, Kyle E. Venous pH can safely replace arterial pH in the initial evaluation of patients in the emergency department. *Emerg Med J*. 2001.

25. Middleton P, Kelly AM, Brown J, Robertson M. Agreement between arterial and central venous values for pH, bicarbonate,

base excess, and lactate. *Emerg Med J.* 2006.

26. Koul P, Khan U, Wani A, et al. Comparison and agreement between venous and arterial gas analysis in cardiopulmonary patients in Kashmir valley of the Indian subcontinent. *Ann Thorac Med.* 2011.

27. Awasthi S, Rani R, Malviya D. Peripheral venous blood gas analysis: An alternative to arterial blood gas analysis for initial assessment and resuscitation in emergency and intensive care unit patients. *Anesth essays Res.* 2013.

28. Treger R, Pirouz S, Kamangar N, Corry D. Agreement between Central Venous and Arterial Blood Gas Measurements in the Intensive Care Unit. *Clin J Am Soc Nephrol.* 2010.

29. Yildizdaş D, Yapicioğlu H, Yilmaz HL, Sertdemir Y. Correlation of simultaneously obtained capillary, venous, and arterial blood gases of patients in a paediatric intensive care unit. *Arch Dis Child.* 2004.

30. Hynes D, Bates S, Loughman A, Klim S, French C, Kelly AM. Arteriovenous blood gas agreement in intensive care patients with varying levels of circulatory compromise: A pilot study. *C Care Resusc.* 2015.

31. Ma OJ, Rush MD, Godfrey MM, Gaddis G. Arterial blood gas results rarely influence emergency physician management of patients with suspected diabetic ketoacidosis. *Acad Emerg Me* 2003.

32. Zaouter C, Zavorsky GS. The measurement of carboxyhemoglobin and methemoglobin using a non-invasive

pulse CO-oximeter. *Respir Physiol Neurobiol*. 2012;182(2-3):88-92.

33. Touger M, Gallagher EJ, Tyrell J. Relationship Between Venous and Arterial Carboxyhemoglobin Levels in Patients With Suspected Carbon Monoxide Poisoning. *Ann Emerg Med*. 1995;25(4):481-483.

34. Schriger DL, Larmon B, LeGassick T, Blinman T. Spinal immobilization on a flat backboard: does it result in neutral position of the cervical spine? *Ann Emerg Med*. 1991;20(8):878-881.

35. Richards D, Carhart M, Raasch C, Pierce J, Steffey D, Ostarello A. Incidence of thoracic and lumbar spine injuries for restrained occupants in frontal collisions. *Annu proceedings Assoc Adv Automot Med*. 2006;50:125-139.

36. Wampler DA, Pineda C, Polk J, et al. The long spine board does not reduce lateral motion during transport--a randomized healthy volunteer crossover trial. *Am J Emerg Med*. 2016;34(4):717-721.

37. Engsberg JR, Standeven JW, Shurtleff TL, Eggars JL, Shafer JS, Naunheim RS. Cervical spine motion during extrication. *J Emerg Med*. 2013;44(1):122-127.

38. Hauswald M, Ong G, Tandberg D, Omar Z. Out-of-hospital spinal immobilization: its effect on neurologic injury. *Acad Emerg Med*. 1998;5(3):214-219.

39. White CC, Domeier RM, Millin MG, Standards and Clinical Practice Committee NA of EP. EMS spinal precautions and the

use of the long backboard - resource document to the position
statement of the National Association of EMS Physicians and the
American College of Surgeons Committee on Trauma. *Prehosp
Emerg Care*. 2013;18(2):306-314.

40. Baumchen J, Gurss E, Hennes E, Nyberg S, Berg-copas GM. Near
Infrared Spectroscopy Measurement of Sacral Tissue
Oxygenation Saturation (StO 2) in Healthy Volunteers
Immobilized on Spine Boards. *Am J Phys Med*. 2009:76-77.

41. The American College of Surgeons. Advanced trauma life support
(ATLS). *J Trauma Acute Care Surg*. 1985;4:1-392.

42. Poulton TJ. ATLS paradigm fails. *Ann Emerg Med*.
1988;17(1):107.

43. Deakin CD. Accuracy of the advanced trauma life support
guidelines for predicting systolic blood pressure using carotid,
femoral, and radial pulses: observational study. *Bmj*.
2000;321(7262):673-674.

44. McManus J, Yershov AL, Ludwig D, et al. Radial pulse character
relationships to systolic blood pressure and trauma outcomes.
Prehospital Emerg Care. 2005;9(4):423-428.

45. Manley G, Knudson MM, Morabito D, Damron S, Erickson V, Pitts
L. Hypotension, hypoxia, and head injury: frequency, duration,
and consequences. *Arch Surg*. 2001;136(10):1118-1123.

46. Spaite DW, Hu C, Bobrow BJ, et al. Mortality and prehospital
blood pressure in patients with major traumatic brain injury:
Implications for the hypotension threshold. *JAMA Surg*.
2017;152(4):360-368.

47. Rao P, Knaus EE. Evolution of nonsteroidal anti-inflammatory drugs (NSAIDs): cyclooxygenase (COX) inhibition and beyond. *J Pharm Pharm Sci*. 2008;11(2):81s-110s.

48. Pountos I, Georgouli T, Calori GM, Giannoudis P V. Do nonsteroidal anti-inflammatory drugs affect bone healing? A critical analysis. *ScientificWorldJournal*. 2012;2012.

49. Zhang X, Schwarz EM, Young DA, Puzas JE, Rosier RN, O'Keefe RJ. Cyclooxygenase-2 regulates mesenchymal cell differentiation into the osteoblast lineage and is critically involved in bone repair. *J Clin Invest*. 2002;109(11):1405-1415.

50. Lin CH, Jee WSS, Ma YF, Setterberg RB. Early effects of prostaglandin E2 on bone formation and resorption in different bone sites of rats. *Bone*. 1995;17(4 SUPPL.).

51. Jee WSS, Ueno K, Deng YP, Woodbury DM. The effects of prostaglandin E2 in growing rats: Increased metaphyseal hard tissue and cortico-endosteal bone formation. *Calcif Tissue Int*. 1985;37(2):148-157.

52. Drendel AL, Gorelick MH, Weisman SJ, Lyon R, Brousseau DC, Kim MK. A Randomized Clinical Trial of Ibuprofen Versus Acetaminophen With Codeine for Acute Pediatric Arm Fracture Pain. *Ann Emerg Med*. 2009;54(4):553-560.

53. Chang AK, Bijur PE, Esses D, Barnaby DP, Baer J. Effect of a single dose of oral opioid and nonopioid analgesics on acute extremity pain in the emergency department: A randomized clinical trial. *JAMA - J Am Med Assoc*. 2017;318(17):1661-1667.

54. Borgeat A, Ofner C, Saporito A, Farshad M, Aguirre J. The effect

of nonsteroidal anti-inflammatory drugs on bone healing in humans: A qualitative, systematic review. *J Clin Anesth.* 2018;49(May):92-100.

55. Adolphson P, Abbaszadegan H, Jonsson U, Dalén N, Sjöberg HE, Kalén S. No effects of piroxicam on osteopenia and recovery after Colles' fracture - A randomized, double-blind, placebo-controlled, prospective trial. *Arch Orthop Trauma Surg.* 1993;112(3):127-130.

56. Burd TA, Hughes MS, Anglen JO. Heterotopic ossification prophylaxis with indomethacin increases the risk of long-bone nonunion. *J bone Jt Surg Br Vol.* 2003;85(5):700-705.

57. Sagi HC, Jordan CJ, Barei DP, Serrano-Riera R, Steverson B. Indomethacin prophylaxis for heterotopic ossification after acetabular fracture surgery increases the risk for nonunion of the posterior wall. *J Orthop Trauma.* 2014;28(7):377-383.

58. DePeter KC, Blumberg SM, Dienstag Becker S, Meltzer JA. Does the Use of Ibuprofen in Children with Extremity Fractures Increase their Risk for Bone Healing Complications? *J Emerg Med.* 2017;52(4):426-432.

59. Kay RM, Directo MP, Leathers M, Myung K, Skaggs DL. Complications of ketorolac use in children undergoing operative fracture care. *J Pediatr Orthop.* 2010;30(7):655-658.

60. Marquez-Lara A, Hutchinson ID, Nuñez F, Smith TL, Miller AN. Nonsteroidal anti-inflammatory drugs and bone-healing: A systematic review of research quality. *JBJS Rev.* 2016;4(3):1-14.

61. Dodwell ER, Latorre JG, Parisini E, et al. NSAID exposure and ri

of nonunion: A meta-analysis of case-control and cohort studies. *Calcif Tissue Int.* 2010;87(3):193-202.

62. Walter FG, Gibly RL, Knopp RK, Roe DJ. Squamous cells as predictors of bacterial contamination in urine samples. *Ann Emerg Med.* 1998;31(4):455-458.

63. Mohr NM, Harland KK, Crabb V, et al. Urinary Squamous Epithelial Cells Do Not Accurately Predict Urine Culture Contamination, but May Predict Urinalysis Performance in Predicting Bacteriuria. Zehtabchi S, ed. *Acad Emerg Med.* 2016;23(3):323-330.

64. Kass EH, Finland M. Asymptomatic infections of the urinary tract. *J Urol.* 2002;168(2):420-424.

65. Smith PJ, Morris AJ, Reller LB. Predicting urine culture results by dipstick testing and phase contrast microscopy. *Pathology.* 2003.

66. Curley GF. Rapid sequence induction with rocuronium - a challenge to the gold standard. *Crit Care.* 2011;15(5):9-10.

67. Levine M, Brown DFM. Succinylcholine-induced hyperkalemia in a patient with multiple sclerosis. *J Emerg Med.* 2012;43(2):279-282.

68. Ording H. Incidence of malignant hyperthermia in Denmark. *Anesth Analg.* 1985;64(7):700-704.

69. Sluga M, Ummenhofer W, Studer W, Siegemund M, Marsch SC. Rocuronium versus succinylcholine for rapid sequence induction of anesthesia and endotracheal intubation: A prospective, randomized trial in emergent cases. *Anesth Analg.* 2005;101(5):1356-1361.

70. Patanwala AE, Stahle SA, Sakles JC, Erstad BL. Comparison of succinylcholine and rocuronium for first-attempt intubation success in the emergency department. *Acad Emerg Med.* 2011;18(1):11-14.

71. Wright PMC, Caldwell JE, Miller RD. Onset and duration of rocuronium and succinylcholine at the adductor pollicis and laryngeal adductor muscles in anesthetized humans. *Anesthesiology.* 1994;81(5):1110-1115.

72. Karcioglu O, Arnold J, Topacoglu H, Ozucelik DN, Kiran S, Sonm N. Succinylcholine or rocuronium? A meta-analysis of the effe on intubation conditions. *Int J Clin Pract.* 2006;60(12):1638-1646.

73. Jj P, Js L, Vah S, et al. Rocuronium versus succinylcholine for rapid sequence induction intubation (Review) Rocuronium versus succinylcholine for rapid sequence induction intubation *Victoria.* 2008;(2):2-4.

74. Thiel B, Sarau A, Ng D. Efficacy of Topical Analgesics in Pain Control for Corneal Abrasions: A Systematic Review. *Cureus.* 2017.

75. The New England Journal of Medicine Downloaded from nejm.org at UTSA Libraries on November 21, 2015. For person use only. No other uses without permission. From the NEJM Archive. Copyright © 2010 Massachusetts Medical Society. All rights reserved. 2010.

76. Pharmakakis NM, Katsimpris JM, Melachrinou MP, Koliopoulo JX. Corneal complications following abuse of topical anestheti

Eur J Ophthalmol. 2002;12(5):373-378.

77. Rosenwasser GOD, Holland S, Pflugfelder SC, et al. Topical Anesthetic Abuse. *Ophthalmology.* 1990.

78. Ting JYS, Barns KJ, Holmes JL. Management of Ocular Trauma in Emergency (MOTE) Trial: A pilot randomized double-blinded trial comparing topical amethocaine with saline in the outpatient management of corneal trauma. *J emergencies, trauma Shock.* 2009.

79. Ball IM, Seabrook J, Desai N, Allen L, Anderson S. Dilute proparacaine for the management of acute corneal injuries in the emergency department. *Can J Emerg Med.* 2010.

80. Waldman N, Densie IK, Herbison P. Topical tetracaine used for 24 hours is safe and rated highly effective by patients for the treatment of pain caused by corneal abrasions: A double-blind, randomized clinical trial. *Acad Emerg Med.* 2014.

81. Waldman N, Winrow B, Densie I, et al. An Observational Study to Determine Whether Routinely Sending Patients Home With a 24-Hour Supply of Topical Tetracaine From the Emergency Department for Simple Corneal Abrasion Pain Is Potentially Safe. *Ann Emerg Med.* 2018.

82. Schlosser RJ. Epistaxis. *N Engl J Med.* 2009;360(8):784-789.

83. Min HJ, Kang H, Choi GJ, Kim KS. Association between Hypertension and Epistaxis: Systematic Review and Meta-analysis. *Otolaryngol Neck Surg.* 2017:019459981772144.

84. Riseman JEF, Weiss S. The symptomatology of arterial hypertension. *Am J Med Sci.* 1930;180(1):47-58.

85. Ibrashi F, Sabri N, Eldawi M, Belal A. Effect of atherosclerosis a hypertension on arterial epistaxis. *J Laryngol Otol*. 1978.

86. Fuchs FD, Moreira LB, Pires CP, et al. Absence of association between hypertension and epistaxis: A population-based stud *Blood Press*. 2003;12(3):145-148.

87. Ando Y, Iimura J, Arai S, et al. Risk factors for recurrent epistax Importance of initial treatment. *Auris Nasus Larynx*. 2014.

88. Khan M, Conroy K, Ubayasiri K, et al. Initial assessment in the management of adult epistaxis: Systematic review. *J Laryngol Otol*. 2017;131(12):1035-1055.

89. Herkner H, Havel C, Müllner M, et al. Active epistaxis at ED presentation is associated with arterial hypertension. *Am J Emerg Med*. 2002;20(2):92-95.

90. Herkner H, Laggner AN, Müllner M, et al. Hypertension in patients presenting with epistaxis. *Ann Emerg Med*. 2000;35(2):126-130.

91. Theodosis P, Mouktaroudi M, Papadogiannis D, Ladas S, Papaspyrou S. Epistaxis of patients admitted in the emergency department is not indicative of underlying arterial hypertensic *Rhinology*. 2009.

92. Isezuo SA, Segun-Busari S, Ezunu E, et al. Relationship betwee epistaxis and hypertension: A study of patients seen in the emergency units of two tertiary health institutions in Nigeria. *Niger J Clin Pract*. 2008.

93. Awan MS, Iqbal M, Imam SZ. Epistaxis: When are coagulation studies justified? *Emerg Med J*. 2008;25(3):156-157.

94.   Kucik CJ, Clenney T. Management of epistaxis. *Am Fam Physician*. 2005;71(2):305-312.

95.   Schlosser RJ. Clinical practice. Epistaxis. *N Engl J Med*. 2009.

96.   Kossuth LC. The removal of injured personnel from wrecked vehicles. *J Trauma - Inj Infect Crit Care*. 1965;5(6):703-708.

97.   Farrington JD. Death in a Ditch. *Bull Am Coll Surg*. 1967;98(6):44.

98.   Podolsky S, Baraff LJ, Simon RR, Hoffman JR, Larmon B, Ablon W. Efficacy of cervical spine immobilization methods. *J Trauma - Inj Infect Crit Care*. 1983;23(6):461-465.

99.   Kwan I, Bunn F, Roberts IG. Spinal immobilisation for trauma patients. *Cochrane Database Syst Rev*. 2001;(2).

100.   Horodyski M, DiPaola CP, Conrad BP, Rechtine GR. Cervical collars are insufficient for immobilizing an unstable cervical spine injury. *J Emerg Med*. 2011;41(5):513-519.

101.   Dixon M, O'Halloran J, Cummins NM. Biomechanical analysis of spinal immobilisation during prehospital extrication: A proof of concept study. *Emerg Med J*. 2014;31(9):745-749.

102.   Sundstrøm T, Asbjørnsen H, Habiba S, Sunde GA, Wester K. Prehospital Use of Cervical Collars in Trauma Patients: A Critical Review. *J Neurotrauma*. 2014;31(6):531-540.

103.   Ben-Galim P, Dreiangel N, Mattox KL, Reitman CA, Kalantar SB, Hipp JA. Extrication collars can result in abnormal separation between vertebrae in the presence of a dissociative injury. *J Trauma - Inj Infect Crit Care*. 2010;69(2):447-450.

104.   Walters BC, Hadley MN, Hurlbert RJ, et al. Guidelines for the Management of Acute Cervical Spine and Spinal Cord Injuries.

Neurosurgery. 2013;60:82-91.

105. Kanji S, MacLean RD. Cardiac Glycoside Toxicity. More Than 20 Years and Counting. *Crit Care Clin*. 2012;28(4):527-535.

106. Levine M, Nikkanen H, Pallin DJ. The effects of intravenous calcium in patients with digoxin toxicity. *J Emerg Med*. 2011;40(1):41-46.

107. Erickson CP, Olson KR. Case files of the medical toxicology fellowship of the California poison control system-San Francisco calcium plus digoxin-more taboo than toxic? *J Med Toxicol*. 2008;4(1):33-39.

108. Bower JO, Mengle HAK. The additive effect of calcium and digitalis: A warning, with a report of two deaths. *J Am Med Assoc*. 1936;106(14):1151-1153.

109. Shrager MW. Digitalis Intoxication: A Review and Report of Four Cases, with Emphasis on Etiology. *AMA Arch Intern Med*. 1957;100(6):881-893.

110. Nola GT, Pope S, Harrison DC. Assessment of the synergistic relationship between serum calcium and digitalis. *Am Heart J*. 1970;79(4):499-507.

111. Hack JB, Woody JH, Lewis DE, Brewer K, Meggs WJ. The effect calcium chloride in treating hyperkalemia due to acute digoxin toxicity in a porcine model. *J Toxicol - Clin Toxicol*. 2004;42(4):337-342.

112. Van Deusen SK, Birkhahn RH, Gaeta TJ. Treatment of hyperkalemia in a patient with unrecognized digitalis toxicity. *Toxicol - Clin Toxicol*. 2003;41(4):373-376.

113. Fenton F, Smally AJ, Laut J. Hyperkalemia and digoxin toxicity in a patient with kidney failure. *Ann Emerg Med*. 1996;28(4):440-441.

114. Paradis NA, Koscove EM. Epinephrine in cardiac arrest: a critical review. *Ann Emerg Med*. 1990;19(11):1288-1301.

115. Gough CJR, Nolan JP. The role of adrenaline in cardiopulmonary resuscitation. *Crit Care*. 2018;22(1):139.

116. Link MS, Berkow LC, Kudenchuk PJ, et al. Part 7: Adult advanced cardiovascular life support: 2015 American Heart Association guidelines update for cardiopulmonary resuscitation and emergency cardiovascular care. *Circulation*. 2015;132(18):S444-S464.

117. Nakahara S, Tomio J, Takahashi H, et al. Evaluation of pre-hospital administration of adrenaline (epinephrine) by emergency medical services for patients with out of hospital cardiac arrest in Japan: controlled propensity matched retrospective cohort study. *BMJ*. 2013;347(December):f6829.

118. Goto YYN, Maeda T, Goto YYN. Effects of prehospital epinephrine during out-of-hospital cardiac arrest with initial non-shockable rhythm: an observational cohort study. *Crit Care*. 2013;17(5):R188.

119. Hagihara A, Hasegawa M, Abe T, Nagata T, Wakata Y, Miyazaki S. Prehospital Epinephrine Use and Survival Among Patients With Out-of-Hospital Cardiac Arrest. *Jama*. 2012;307(11):1161.

120. Loomba RS, Nijhawan K, Aggarwal S, Arora RR. Increased return of spontaneous circulation at the expense of neurologic

outcomes: Is prehospital epinephrine for out-of-hospital cardia arrest really worth it? *J Crit Care*. 2015;30(6):1376-1381.

121. &NA; Intravenous Drug Administration During Out-of-Hospital Cardiac Arrest. *Surv Anesthesiol*. 2010;54(5):256-257.

122. Perkins GD, Ji C, Deakin CD, et al. A Randomized Trial of Epinephrine in Out-of-Hospital Cardiac Arrest. *N Engl J Med*. 2018:NEJMoa1806842.

123. Cowley RA, Demetriades A, Mansberger AR, Attar S, Esmond WG, Bessman S. Hemorrhagic shock in dogs treated with extracorporeal circulation. A study of survival time and blood chemistry levels. *Surg Forum*. 1960;11:110-112.

124. Center U of MM. History of the Shock Trauma Center.

125. Franklin J, Doelp A. *Shock-Trauma*. 1st ed. Martin's Press; 198

126. Dutton RP. Shock and trauma anesthesia. *Anesthesiol Clin Nor America*. 1999;17(1):83-95.

127. Siegel JH. Posttrauma Oxygen Debt and Its Metabolic Consequences. In: *Anaesthesia, Pain, Intensive Care and Emergency Medicine — A.P.I.C.E.* Milano: Springer Milan; 1996:225-233.

128. Kendall McNabney W. Vietnam in context. *Ann Emerg Med*. 1981;10(12):659-661.

129. Santy P, Moulinier M, Marquis D. *Shock Tramatique Dans Les Blessures de Guerre, Analysis d'observations*. Vol 44.; 1918.

130. Feero S, Hedges JR, Simmons E, Irwin L. Does out-of-hospital EMS time affect trauma survival? *Am J Emerg Med*. 1995;13(2):133-135.

131. Lerner EB, Moscati RM. The Golden Hour: Scientific Fact or Medical "Urban Legend"? *Acad Emerg Med*. 2001;8(7):758-760.

132. Bledsoe BE. The Golden Hour: fact or fiction? *Emerg Med Serv*. 2002;31(6):105.

133. Nöske HD, Kraus SW, Altinkilic BM, Weidner W. Historical milestones regarding torsion of the scrotal organs. *J Urol*. 1998;159(1):13-16.

134. Lauenstein C. *Die Torsion Des Hodens*. Druck und Verlag von Breitkopf und Härtel; 1894.

135. Ombredanne L. Torsions testiculaires chez les enfants. *Bull Mem Soc Chir*. 1913;38:779.

136. Rabinowitz R. The importance of the cremasteric reflex in acute scrotal swelling in children. *J Urol*. 1984;132(1):89-90.

137. Kadish HA, Bolte RG. A retrospective review of pediatric patients with epididymitis, testicular torsion, and torsion of testicular appendages. *Pediatrics*. 1998;102(1 Pt 1):73-76.

138. Caldamone AA, Valvo JR, Altebarmakian VK, Rabinowitz R. Acute scrotal swelling in children. *J Pediatr Surg*. 1984;19(5):581-584.

139. Lyronis ID, Ploumis N, Vlahakis I, Charissis G. Acute scrotum - etiology, clinical presentation and seasonal variation. *Indian J Pediatr*. 2009;76(4):407-410.

140. Bingöl-Koloğlu M, Tanyel FC, Anlar B, Büyükpamukçu N. Cremasteric reflex and retraction of a testis. *J Pediatr Surg*. 2001;36(6):863-867.

141. Van Glabeke E, Khairouni A, Larroquet M, Audry G, Gruner M. Acute scrotal pain in children: Results of 543 surgical

explorations. *Pediatr Surg Int*. 1999;15(5-6):353-357.

142. Beni-Israel T, Goldman M, Bar Chaim S, Kozer E. Clinical predictors for testicular torsion as seen in the pediatric ED. *An Emerg Med*. 2010;28(7):786-789.

143. Murphy FL, Fletcher L, Pease P. Early scrotal exploration in all cases is the investigation and intervention of choice in the acu paediatric scrotum. *Pediatr Surg Int*. 2006;22(5):413-416.

144. Ciftci AO, Şenocak ME, Cahit Tanyel F, Büyükpamukçu N. Clini predictors for differential diagnosis of acute scrotum. *Eur J Pediatr Surg*. 2004;14(5):333-338.

145. Karmazyn B, Steinberg R, Kornreich L, et al. Clinical and sonographic criteria of acute scrotum in children: A retrospect study of 172 boys. *Pediatr Radiol*. 2005;35(3):302-310.

146. Eaton SH, Cendron MA, Estrada CR, et al. Intermittent testicul torsion: Diagnostic features and management outcomes. *J Ur* 2005;174(4 II):1532-1535.

147. Waldert M, Klatte T, Schmidbauer J, Remzi M, Lackner J, Marberger M. Color Doppler Sonography Reliably Identifies Testicular Torsion in Boys. *Urology*. 2010;75(5):1170-1174.

148. LB M. Torsion of the testicle: it is time to stop tossing the dice *Pediatr Emerg Care*. 2012;28(1):80-86.

149. Gerardi MJ, Sacchetti AD, Cantor RM, et al. Rapid-sequence intubation of the pediatric patient. Pediatric Emergency Medicine Committee of the American College of Emergency Physicians. *Ann Emerg Med*. 1996;28(1):55-74.

150. Leigh MD, McCoy DD, Belton MK, Lewis GB. Bradycardia

following intravenous administration of succinylcholine chloride to infants and children. *Anesthesiology*. 2018;18(5):698-702.

151. Lupprian KG, Churchill-Davidson HC. Effect of suxamethonium on cardiac rhythm. *Br Med J*. 1960;2(5215):1774-1777.

152. Green DW, Bristow ASE, Fisher M. Comparison of I.V. Glycopyrrolate and atropine in the prevention of bradycardia and arrhythmias following repeated doses of suxamethonium in children. *Br J Anaesth*. 1984;56(9):981-985.

153. MATHIAS JA, EVANS-PROSSER CDG, CHURCHILL-DAVIDSON HC. the Role of the Non-Depolarizing Drugs in the Prevention of Suxamethonium Bradycardia. *Br J Anaesth*. 1970;42(7):609-613.

154. Cordero L, Hon EH. Neonatal bradycardia following nasopharyngeal stimulation. *J Pediatr*. 1971;78(3):441-447.

155. Development C, Development C. Autonomic Function in the Neonate : VII . Maturational Changes in Cardiac Control Author (s): Earle L . Lipton , Alfred Steinschneider and Julius B . Richmond Published by : Wiley on behalf of the Society for Research in Child Development Stable URL : h. 2019;37(1):1-16.

156. Goudsouzian NG. Mivacurium in infants and children. *Paediatr Anaesth*. 1997;7(3):183-190.

157. Guyton DC, Scharf SM. Should atropine be routine in children? *Can J Anaesth*. 1996;43(7):754-755.

158. Joulia F, Lemaitre F, Fontanari P, Mille ML, Barthelemy P. Circulatory effects of apnoea in elite breath-hold divers. *Acta Physiol*. 2009;197(1):75-82.

159. McAuliffe G, Bissonnette B, Boutin C. Should the routine use of

atropine before succinylcholine in children be reconsidered? C

J Anaesth. 1995;42(8):724-729.

160. Fastle RK, Roback MG. Incidence of Reflex Bradycardia and

Effects. *Pediatr Emerg Care.* 2004;20(10):651-655.

161. Jones P, Dauger S, Peters MJ. Bradycardia during critical care

intubation: Mechanisms, significance and atropine. *Arch Dis

Child.* 2012;97(2):139-144.

162. Adams RG, Verma P, Jackson AJ, Miller RL. Plasma

pharmacokinetics of intravenously administered atropine in

normal human subjects. *J Clin Pharmacol.* 1982;22(10):477-48

163. Magbagbeola JAO. The effect of atropine premedication on bc

temperature of children in the tropics. *Br J Anaesth.*

1973;45(11):1139-1142.

164. Shehadi WH. Adverse reactions to intravascularly administere

contrast media. A comprehensive study based on a prospectiv

survey. *Am J Roentgenol Radium Ther Nucl Med.*

1975;124(1):145-152.

165. Beaty AD, Lieberman PL, Slavin RG. Seafood allergy and

radiocontrast media: are physicians propagating a myth? *Am

Med.* 2008;121(2):158.e1-4.

166. Schabelman E, Witting M. The relationship of radiocontrast,

iodine, and seafood allergies: A medical myth exposed. *J Eme

Med.* 2010;39(5):701-707.

167. Media AC on D and C. *ACR Manual on Contrast Media.*; 2018.

168. Lasser EC, Lyon SG, Berry CC. Reports on contrast media

reactions: analysis of data from reports to the U.S. Food and

Drug Administration. *Radiology*. 1997;203(3):605-610.

169. Katayama H, Yamaguchi K, Kozuka T, Takashima T, Seez P, Matsuura K. Adverse reactions to ionic and nonionic contrast media. A report from the Japanese Committee on the Safety of Contrast Media. *Radiology*. 1990;175(3):621-628.

170. Assimos D, Krambeck A, Miller NL, et al. Surgical Management of Stones: American Urological Association/Endourological Society Guideline, PART I. *J Urol*. 2016;196(4):1153-1160.

171. Türk C, Petřík A, Sarica K, et al. EAU Guidelines on Diagnosis and Conservative Management of Urolithiasis. *Eur Urol*. 2016;69(3):468-474.

172. Hollingsworth JM, Canales BK, Rogers MAM, et al. Alpha blockers for treatment of ureteric stones: Systematic review and meta-analysis. *BMJ*. 2016;355.

173. Singh A, Alter HJ, Littlepage A. A Systematic Review of Medical Therapy to Facilitate Passage of Ureteral Calculi. *Ann Emerg Med*. 2007;50(5):552-563.

174. Campschroer T, Zhu Y, Duijvesz D, Grobbee DE, Lock MTWT. Alpha-blockers as medical expulsive therapy for ureteral stones. *Cochrane Database Syst Rev*. 2014;2014(4).

175. Seitz C, Liatsikos E, Porpiglia F, Tiselius HG, Zwergel U. Medical Therapy to Facilitate the Passage of Stones: What Is the Evidence? *Eur Urol*. 2009;56(3):455-471.

176. Pickard R, Starr K, MacLennan G, et al. Medical expulsive therapy in adults with ureteric colic: A multicentre, randomised, placebo-controlled trial. *Lancet*. 2015;386(9991):341-349.

177. Meltzer AC, Burrows PK, Wolfson AB, et al. Effect of Tamsulosin on Passage of Symptomatic Ureteral Stones: A Randomized Clinical Trial. *JAMA Intern Med.* 2018;178(8):1051-1057.

178. Furyk JS, Chu K, Banks C, et al. Distal Ureteric Stones and Tamsulosin: A Double-Blind, Placebo-Controlled, Randomized, Multicenter Trial. *Ann Emerg Med.* 2016;67(1):86-95e2.

179. Wang RC, Smith-Bindman R, Whitaker E, et al. Effect of Tamsulosin on Stone Passage for Ureteral Stones: A Systematic Review and Meta-analysis. *Ann Emerg Med.* 2017;69(3):353-361.e3.

180. Ye Z, Zeng G, Yang H, et al. Efficacy and Safety of Tamsulosin in Medical Expulsive Therapy for Distal Ureteral Stones with Renal Colic: A Multicenter, Randomized, Double-blind, Placebo-controlled Trial. *Eur Urol.* 2017;2(5-6):444-456.

181. Hermanns T, Sauermann P, Rufibach K, Frauenfelder T, Sulser T, Strebel RT. Is There a Role for Tamsulosin in the Treatment of Distal Ureteral Stones of 7 mm or Less? Results of a Randomised, Double-Blind, Placebo-Controlled Trial. *Eur Urol.* 2009;56(3):4-412.

182. Meltzer AC, Burrows PK, Wolfson AB, et al. Effect of Tamsulosin on Passage of Symptomatic Ureteral Stones. *JAMA Intern Med.* 2018;55(5):734-735.

183. Ferre RM, Wasielewski JN, Strout TD, Perron AD. Tamsulosin for Ureteral Stones in the Emergency Department: A Randomized Controlled Trial. *Ann Emerg Med.* 2009;54(3):432-439.e2.

184. Kaplan SA. Side Effects of alpha-Blocker Use: Retrograde

Ejaculation. *Rev Urol.* 2009;11(Suppl 1):S14-8.

185. Kouba DJ, Lopiccolo MC, Alam M, et al. Guidelines for the use of local anesthesia in office-based dermatologic surgery. *J Am Acad Dermatol.* 2016;74(6):1201-1219.

186. Wilhelmi BJ, Blackwell SJ, Miller JH, et al. Do not use epinephrine in digital blocks: Myth or truth? *Plast Reconstr Surg.* 2001;107(2):393-397.

187. Bunnell S. *Surgery of the Hand.* 3rd ed. Philadelphia: Lippincott; 1956.

188. FJ S, Mcgill JW, Goings MA, et al. A precaution in the use of procaine-epinephrine for regional anesthesia. *J Am Med Assoc.* 1928;91(1):43-44.

189. KAUFMAN PA. GANGRENE FOLLOWING DIGITAL NERVE BLOCK ANESTHESIA. *Arch Surg.* 1941;42(5):929.

190. McLaughlin CW. Postoperative gangrene of the finger following digital nerve block anesthesia: Report of a case. *Am J Surg.* 1942;55(3):588-589.

191. Garlock JH. Gangrene of the Finger Following Digital Nerve Block Anaesthesia. *Ann Surg.* 1931;94(6):1103-1107.

192. Ilicki J. Safety of Epinephrine in Digital Nerve Blocks: A Literature Review. *J Emerg Med.* 2015;49(5):799-809.

193. Thomson CJ, Lalonde DH, Denkler KA, Feicht AJ. A critical look at the evidence for and against elective epinephrine use in the finger. *Plast Reconstr Surg.* 2007;119(1):260-266.

194. Muck AE, Bebarta VS, Borys DJ, Morgan DL. Six years of epinephrine digital injections: Absence of significant local or

systemic effects. *Ann Emerg Med*. 2010;56(3):270-274.

195. Nodwell T, Lalonde D. How long does it take phentolamine to reverse adrenaline-induced vasoconstriction in the finger and hand? A prospective, randomized, blinded study: the Dalhousie project experimental phase. *Can J Plast Surg*. 2003;11(4):187-190.

196. Fitzcharles-Bowe C, Denkler K, Lalonde D. Finger injection with high-dose (1:1,000) epinephrine: Does it cause finger necrosis and should it be treated? *Hand*. 2007;2(1):5-11.

197. Hinterberger JW, Kintzi HE. Phentolamine reversal of epinephrine-induced digital vasospasm. How to save an ischemic finger. *Arch Fam Med*. 1994;3(2):193-195.

198. Velissariou I, Cottrell S, Berry K, Wilson B. Management of adrenaline (epinephrine) induced digital ischaemia in children after accidental injection from an EpiPen. *Emerg Med J*. 2004;21(3):387-388.

199. Firoz B, Davis N, Goldberg LH. Local anesthesia using buffered 0.5% lidocaine with 1:200,000 epinephrine for tumors of the digits treated with Mohs micrographic surgery. *J Am Acad Dermatol*. 2009;61(4):639-643.

200. Schnabl SM, Herrmann N, Wilder D, Breuninger H, Häfner H-M. Clinical Results for use of local anesthesia with epinephrine in penile nerve block. *JDDG J der Dtsch Dermatologischen Gesellschaft*. 2014;12(4):332-339.

201. Oosterlinck W, Philp NH, Charig C, Gillies G, Hetherington JW, Lloyd J. A Double-Blind Single Dose Comparison of Intramuscu

Ketorolac Tromethamine and Pethidine in the Treatment of Renal Colic. *J Clin Pharmacol*. 1990;30(4):336-341.

202. Larkin GL, Peacock IV WF, Pearl SM, Blair GA, D'Amico F. Efficacy of ketorolac tromethamine versus meperidine in the ED treatment of acute renal colic. *Am J Emerg Med*. 1999;17(1):6-10.

203. Rainer TH. Cost effectiveness analysis of intravenous ketorolac and morphine for treating pain after limb injury: double blind randomised controlled trial. *Bmj*. 2000;321(7271):1247-1247.

204. POWELL H, SMALLMAN JMB, MORGAN M. Comparison of intramuscular ketorolac and morphine in pain control after laparotomy. *Anaesthesia*. 1990;45(7):538-542.

205. Power I, Noble DW, Douglas E, Spence AA. Comparison of I.M. ketorolac trometamol and morphine sulphate for pain relief after cholecystectomy. *Br J Anaesth*. 1990;65(4):448-455.

206. Spindler JS, Mehlisch D, Brown CR. Intramuscular ketorolac and morphine in the treatment of moderate to severe pain after major surgery. *Pharmacother J Hum Pharmacol Drug Ther*. 1990;10(6P2):51S--58S.

207. Morrison NA, Repka MX. Ketorolac versus Acetaminophen or Ibuprofen in Controlling Postoperative Pain in Patients with Strabismus. *Ophthalmology*. 1994;101(5):915-918.

208. Wright JM, Price SD, Watson WA. NSAID use and efficacy in the emergency department: single doses of oral ibuprofen versus intramuscular ketorolac. *Ann Pharmacother*. 1994;28(3):309-312.

209. Turturro MA, Paris PM, Seaberg DC. Intramuscular Ketorolac Versus Oral Ibuprofen in Acute Musculoskeletal Pain. *Ann Emer Med*. 1995;26(2):117-120.

210. Neighbor ML, Puntillo KA. Intramuscular ketorolac vs oral ibuprofen in emergency department patients with acute pain. *Acad Emerg Med*. 1998;5(2):118-122.

211. Mixter III CG, Meeker LD, Gavin TJ. Preemptive Pain Control in Patients Having Laparoscopic Hernia Repair. *Arch Surg*. 1998;133(4):432-437.

212. Braaten KP, Hurwitz S, Fortin J, Goldberg AB. Intramuscular ketorolac versus oral ibuprofen for pain relief in first-trimester surgical abortion: A randomized clinical trial. *Contraception*. 2014;89(2):116-121.

213. Schwartz NA, Turturro MA, Istvan DJ, Larkin GL. Patients' perceptions of route of nonsteroidal anti-inflammatory drug administration and its effect on analgesia. *Acad Emerg Med*. 2000;7(8):857-861.

214. Massó González EL, Patrignani P, Tacconelli S, García Rodrígue LA. Variability among nonsteroidal antiinflammatory drugs in r of upper gastrointestinal bleeding. *Arthritis Rheum*. 2010;62(6):1592-1601.

215. Lewis SC, Langman MJS, Laporte JR, Matthews JNS, Rawlins M Wiholm BE. Dose-response relationships between individual nonaspirin nonsteroidal anti-inflammatory drugs (NANSAIDs) and serious upper gastrointestinal bleeding: A meta-analysis based on individual patient data. *Br J Clin Pharmacol*.

2002;54(3):320-326.

216. Alberto L, Rodríguez G, Troncon MG. Risk of hospitalization for upper gastrointestinal bleeding associated with ketorolac , other NSAIDs , calcium antagonists and other antihypertensive drugs. *Heal (San Fr.* 1998;158:33-39.

217. Motov S, Yasavolian M, Likourezos A, et al. Comparison of Intravenous Ketorolac at Three Single-Dose Regimens for Treating Acute Pain in the Emergency Department: A Randomized Controlled Trial. *Ann Emerg Med.* 2017;70(2):177-184.

218. Pandit A, Aryal MR, Aryal Pandit A, et al. Preventive PCI versus culprit lesion stenting during primary PCI in acute STMI: A systematic review and meta-analysis. *Open Hear.* 2014;1(1):1-7.

219. Katritsis DG, Ioannidis JPA. Percutaneous coronary intervention versus conservative therapy in nonacute coronary artery disease: A meta-analysis. *Circulation.* 2005;111(22):2906-2912.

220. Boden WE, O'Rourke RA, Teo KK, et al. Optimal medical therapy with or without PCI for stable coronary disease. *N Engl J Med.* 2007;356(15):1503-1516.

221. De Bruyne B, Pijls NHJ, Kalesan B, et al. Fractional Flow Reserve–Guided PCI versus Medical Therapy in Stable Coronary Disease. *N Engl J Med.* 2012;367(11):991-1001.

222. Kinlay S. Quality of life with PCI versus medical therapy in stable coronary disease. *N Engl J Med.* 2008;359(21):2291; author reply 2292.

223. Al-Lamee R, Thompson D, Dehbi HM, et al. Percutaneous

coronary intervention in stable angina (ORBITA): A double-blin randomised controlled trial. *Lancet*. 2017;6736(17):1-11.

224. Freeman R, Wieling W, Axelrod FB, et al. Consensus statement on the definition of orthostatic hypotension, neurally mediated syncope and the postural tachycardia syndrome. *Clin Auton Re* 2011;21(2):69-72.

225. McGee S, Abernethy WB, Simel DL. Is this patient hypovolemic *Am Med Assoc*. 1999;281(11):1022-1029.

226. Schatz IJ, Bannister R, Freeman RL, et al. Consensus statement on the definition of orthostatic hypotension, pure autonomic failure and multiple system atrophy. *Clin Auton Res*. 1996;6(2):125-126.

227. Guidelines P, Review E, Factors LR. Correction to: 2017 ACC/AHA/HRS guideline for the evaluation and management c patients with syncope: Executive summary: A report of the American College of Cardiology/American Heart Association T Force on Clinical Practice Guidelines and the Heart Rhy. *Circulation*. 2017;136(16):e269-e270.

228. Judith E. Tintinalli, J. Stephan Stapczynski DMC, O. John Ma, Ri K. Cydulka GDM. *Tintinalli's Emergency Medicine: A Comprehensive Study Guide*. 8th ed.; 2011.

229. Frith J. Diagnosing orthostatic hypotension: a narrative review the evidence. *Br Med Bull*. 2015;115(1):123-134.

230. Stewart JM. Transient orthostatic hypotension is common in adolescents. *J Pediatr*. 2002;140(4):418-424.

231. Silverstein FE, Gilbert DA, Tedesco FJ, Buenger NK, Persing J. T

National ASGE Survey on Upper Gastrointestinal Bleeding: II. Clinical prognostic factors. *Gastrointest Endosc*. 1981;27(2):80-93.

232. Wu J-S, Lu F-H, Yang Y-C, Chang C-J. Postural Hypotension and Postural Dizziness in Patients With Non–Insulin-Dependent Diabetes. *Arch Intern Med*. 1999;159(12):1350.

233. Laederach-Hofmann K, Weidmann P, Ferrari P. Hypovolemia contributes to the pathogenesis of orthostatic hypotension in patients with diabetes mellitus. *Am J Med*. 1999;106(1):50-58.

234. Ooi WL, Barrett S, Hossain M, Kelley-Gagnon M, Lipsitz LA. Patterns of orthostatic blood pressure change and their clinical correlates in a frail, elderly population. *Jama*. 2015;277(16):1299-1304.

235. Baraff LJ, Schriger DL. Orthostatic Vital Signs : and Sensitivity a 450-mL Blood Loss. *Am J Emerg Med*. 1992;10(2):99-103.

236. Sinert R, Spektor M. Clinical assessment of hypovolemia. *Ann Emerg Med*. 2005;45(3):327-329.

237. Bloom AS, Devlin JJ. Discriminatory Value of Orthostatic Vital Signs in the Emergency Department Evaluation of Syncope. *Ann Emerg Med*. 2017;70(3):438-439.

238. Centers for Disease Control and Prevention (CDC). CDC Grand Rounds: the growing threat of multidrug-resistant gonorrhea. *MMWR Morb Mortal Wkly Rep*. 2013;62(6):103-106.

239. CDC C for DC and P. *CEPHALOSPORIN-RESISTANT NEISSERIA GONORRHOEAE PUBLIC HEALTH RESPONSE PLAN*.; 2012.

240. Workowski KA, Berman S, CDC C for DC and P. Sexually

transmitted diseases treatment guidelines, 2010. *MMWR Recomm Rep*. 2010;59(RR-12):1-110.

241. Moran JS, Levine WC. Drugs of choice for the treatment of uncomplicated gonococcal infections. *Clin Infect Dis*. 1995;20 Suppl 1:S47-65.

242. Bolan GA, Sparling PF, Wasserheit JN. The emerging threat of untreatable gonococcal infection. *N Engl J Med*. 2012;366(6):485-487.

243. Roche. Rocephin (ceftriaxone sodium) for injection.

244. Richards DM, Heel RC, Brogden RN, Speight TM, Avery GS. Ceftriaxone. A review of its antibacterial activity, pharmacological properties and therapeutic use. *Drugs*. 1984;27(6):469-527.

245. Cushing H. The blood pressure reactions of acute cerebral compression, illustrated by cases of intracranial hemorrhage. *J Med Sci*. 1903;125(6):1017–1044.

246. Broderick JP, Adams HP, Barsan W, et al. Guidelines for the Management of Spontaneous Intracerebral Hemorrhage. *Stroke* 1999;30(4):905-915.

247. Anderson CS, Huang Y, Wang JG, et al. Intensive blood pressure reduction in acute cerebral haemorrhage trial (INTERACT): a randomised pilot trial. *Lancet Neurol*. 2008;7(5):391-399.

248. Morgenstern LB, Hemphill JC, Anderson C, et al. Guidelines for the management of spontaneous intracerebral hemorrhage: A guideline for healthcare professionals from the American Heart Association/American Stroke Association. *Stroke*.

2010;41(9):2108-2129.

249. Zazulia AR, Diringer MN, Videen TO, et al. Hypoperfusion without ischemia surrounding acute intracerebral hemorrhage. *J Cereb Blood Flow Metab*. 2001;21(7):804-810.

250. Anderson CS, Heeley E, Huang Y, et al. Rapid Blood-Pressure Lowering in Patients with Acute Intracerebral Hemorrhage. *N Engl J Med*. 2013;368(25):2355-2365.

251. Bath PMW, Lees KR, Schellinger PD, et al. Statistical analysis of the primary outcome in acute stroke trials. *Stroke*. 2012;43(4):1171-1178.

252. Murray GD, Barer D, Choi S, et al. Design and Analysis of Phase III Trials with Ordered Outcome Scales: The Concept of the Sliding Dichotomy. *J Neurotrauma*. 2005;22(5):511-517.

253. Roozenbeek B, Lingsma HF, Perel P, et al. The added value of ordinal analysis in clinical trials: An example in traumatic brain injury. *Crit Care*. 2011;15(3):R127.

254. Qureshi AI, Palesch YY, Barsan WG, et al. Intensive Blood-Pressure Lowering in Patients with Acute Cerebral Hemorrhage. *N Engl J Med*. 2016;375(11):1033-1043.

255. Faine B, Nunge M, Denning G, Nugent A. Implementing evidence-based changes in emergency department treatment: alternative vitamin therapy for alcohol-related illnesses. *Ann Emerg Med*. 2012;59(5):408-412.

256. Flannery AH, Adkins DA, Cook AM. Unpeeling the Evidence for the Banana Bag: Evidence-Based Recommendations for the Management of Alcohol-Associated Vitamin and Electrolyte

Deficiencies in the ICU. *Crit Care Med.* 2016;44(8):1545-1552.

257. Li SF, Jacob J, Feng J, Kulkarni M. Vitamin deficiencies in acutely intoxicated patients in the ED. *Am J Emerg Med.* 2008;26(7):79 795.

258. Thomson AD, Cook CCH, Touquet R, Henry JA, Royal College of Physicians L. The Royal College of Physicians report on alcohol: guidelines for managing Wernicke's encephalopathy in the accident and Emergency Department. *Alcohol Alcohol.* 2002;37(6):513-521.

259. Faine B, Denning G, Nugent A, Nunge M. In reply. *Ann Emerg Med.* 2013;61(1):120.

260. Sarai M, Tejani AM, Chan AHW, Kuo IF, Li J. Magnesium for alcohol withdrawal. *Cochrane database Syst Rev.* 2013;(6):CD008358.

261. Perez SRS, Keijzers G, Steele M, Byrnes J, Scuffham PA. Intravenous 0.9% sodium chloride therapy does not reduce length of stay of alcohol-intoxicated patients in the emergency department: a randomised controlled trial. *Emerg Med Australas.* 2013;25(6):527-534.

262. Hauck FR, Tanabe KO. Beyond "Back to Sleep": Ways to Further Reduce the Risk of Sudden Infant Death Syndrome. *Pediatr An.* 2017;46(8):e284-e290.

263. Schaefer GR, Matus H, Schumann JH, et al. Financial responsibility of hospitalized patients who left against medical advice: medical urban legend? *J Gen Intern Med.* 2012;27(7):825-830.

264. Wigder HN, Propp DA, Leslie K, Mathew A. Insurance Companies Refusing Payment for Patients Who Leave the Emergency Department Against Medical Advice is a Myth. *Ann Emerg Med*. 2010;55(4):393.

265. Meltzer D, Manning WG, Morrison J, et al. Effects of physician experience on costs and outcomes on an academic general medicine service: results of a trial of hospitalists. *Ann Intern Med*. 2002;137(11):866-874.

266. Bouma GJ, Muizelaar JP, Choi SC, Newlon PG, Young HF. Cerebral circulation and metabolism after severe traumatic brain injury: the elusive role of ischemia. *J Neurosurg*. 1991;75(5):685-693.

267. Steiner LA, Coles JP, Johnston AJ, et al. Responses of Posttraumatic Pericontusional Cerebral Blood Flow and Blood Volume to an Increase in Cerebral Perfusion Pressure. *J Cereb Blood Flow Metab*. 2003;23(11):1371-1377.

268. Gibbs JM. The effect of intravenous ketamine on cerebrospinal fluid pressure. *Br J Anaesth*. 1972;44(12):1298-1302.

269. Shaprio HM, Wyte SR, Harris AB. Ketamine anaesthesia in patients with intracranial pathology. *Br J Anaesth*. 1972;44(11):1200-1204.

270. Wyte SR, Shapiro HM, Turner P, Harris AB. Ketamine-induced intracranial hypertension. *Anesthesiology*. 1972;36(2):174-176.

271. Gardner AE, Dannemiller FJ, Dean D. Intracranial cerebrospinal fluid pressure in man during ketamine anesthesia. *Anesth Analg*. 1972;51(5):741-745.

272. List WF, Crumrine RS, Cascorbi HF, Weiss MH. Increased

cerebrospinal fluid pressure after ketamine. *Anesthesiology*. 1972;36(1):98-99.

273. Bourgoin A, Albanèse J, Léone M, Sampol-Manos E, Viviand X, Martin C. Effects of sufentanil or ketamine administered in target-controlled infusion on the cerebral hemodynamics of severely brain-injured patients. *Crit Care Med*. 2005;33(5):110 1113.

274. Bourgoin A, Albanèse J, Wereszczynski N, Charbit M, Vialet R, Martin C. Safety of sedation with ketamine in severe head injⷡ patients: comparison with sufentanil. *Crit Care Med*. 2003;31(3):711-717.

275. Kolenda H, Gremmelt A, Rading S, Braun U, Markakis E. Ketamine for analgosedative therapy in intensive care treatmɛ of head-injured patients. *Acta Neurochir (Wien)*. 1996;138(10):1193-1199.

276. Albanèse J, Arnaud S, Rey M, Thomachot L, Alliez B, Martin C. Ketamine decreases intracranial pressure and electroencephalographic activity in traumatic brain injury patients during propofol sedation. *Anesthesiology*. 1997;87(6):1328-1334.

277. Mayberg TS, Lam AM, Matta BF, Domino KB, Winn HR. Ketamɨ does not increase cerebral blood flow velocity or intracranial pressure during isoflurane/nitrous oxide anesthesia in patient undergoing craniotomy. *Anesth Analg*. 1995;81(1):84-89.

278. Stahel PF, Smith WR, Moore EE. Hypoxia and hypotension, thɛ "lethal duo" in traumatic brain injury: implications for

prehospital care. *Intensive Care Med*. 2008;34(3):402-404.

279. Alqurashi W, Ellis AK. Do Corticosteroids Prevent Biphasic Anaphylaxis? *J Allergy Clin Immunol Pract*. 2017;5(5):1194-1205.

280. Reber LL, Hernandez JD, Galli SJ. The pathophysiology of anaphylaxis. *J Allergy Clin Immunol*. 2017;140(2):335-348.

281. Anagnostou K, Turner PJ. Myths, facts and controversies in the diagnosis and management of anaphylaxis. *Arch Dis Child*. 2018:83-90.

282. Choo KJL, Simons E, Sheikh A. Glucocorticoids for the treatment of anaphylaxis: Cochrane systematic review. *Allergy Eur J Allergy Clin Immunol*. 2010;65(10):1205-1211.

283. Abaya R, Jones L, Zorc JJ. Dexamethasone Compared to Prednisone for the Treatment of Children with Acute Asthma Exacerbations. *Pediatr Emerg Care*. 2018;34(1):53-60.

284. Charmandari E, Johnston A, Brook CGD, Hindmarsh PC. Bioavailability of oral hydrocortisone in patients with congenital adrenal hyperplasia due to 21-hydroxylase deficiency. *J Endocrinol*. 2001;169(1):65-70.

285. Lieberman P, Nicklas RA, Randolph C, et al. Anaphylaxis—a practice parameter update 2015. *Ann Allergy, Asthma Immunol*. 2015;115(5):341-384.

286. Brown SGA, Stone SF, Fatovich DM, et al. Anaphylaxis: Clinical patterns, mediator release, and severity. *J Allergy Clin Immunol*. 2013;132(5).

287. Lee S, Bellolio MF, Hess EP, Erwin P, Murad MH, Campbell RL. Time of Onset and Predictors of Biphasic Anaphylactic Reactions:

A Systematic Review and Meta-analysis. *J Allergy Clin Immuno* *Pract*. 2015;3(3):408-416.e2.

288. Hochstadter E, Clarke A, De Schryver S, et al. Increasing visits f anaphylaxis and the benefits of early epinephrine administration: A 4-year study at a pediatric emergency department in Montreal, Canada. *J Allergy Clin Immunol*. 2016;137(6):1888-1890.e4.

289. Fleming JT, Clark S, Camargo CA, Rudders SA. Early treatment food-induced anaphylaxis with epinephrine is associated with lower risk of hospitalization. *J Allergy Clin Immunol Pract*. 2015;3(1):57-62.

290. Ellis AK. Priority role of epinephrine in anaphylaxis further underscored--the impact on biphasic anaphylaxis. *Ann Allergy Asthma Immunol*. 2015;115(3):165.

291. Ellis AK, Day JH. Incidence and characteristics of biphasic anaphylaxis: A prospective evaluation of 103 patients. *Ann Allergy, Asthma Immunol*. 2007;98(1):64-69.

292. Michelson KA, Monuteaux MC, Neuman MI. Glucocorticoids a Hospital Length of Stay for Children with Anaphylaxis: A Retrospective Study. *J Pediatr*. 2015;167(3):719-724.e3.

293. Brazil E, MacNamara AF. "Not so immediate" hypersensitivity- the danger of biphasic anaphylactic reactions. *Emerg Med J*. 2008;15(4):252-253.

294. Alqurashi W, Stiell I, Chan K, Neto G, Alsadoon A, Wells G. Epidemiology and clinical predictors of biphasic reactions in children with anaphylaxis. *Ann Allergy, Asthma Immunol*.

2015;115(3):217-223.e2.

295. Mehr S, Liew WK, Tey D, Tang MLK. Clinical predictors for biphasic reactions in children presenting with anaphylaxis. *Clin Exp Allergy*. 2009;39(9):1390-1396.

296. Oya S, Nakamori T, Kinoshita H. Incidence and characteristics of biphasic and protracted anaphylaxis: evaluation of 114 inpatients. *Acute Med Surg*. 2014;1(4):228-233.

297. Sricharoen P, Sittichanbuncha Y, Wibulpolprasert A, Srabongkosh E, Sawanyawisuth K. What clinical factors are associated with biphasic anaphylaxis in Thai adult patients? *Asian Pacific J Allergy Immunol*. 2015;33(1):8-13.

298. D. L, A. A, L. W, et al. A practical guide to the monitoring and management of the complications of systemic corticosteroid therapy. *Allergy, Asthma Clin Immunol*. 2013;9(1):1-25.

299. Nyberg DA, Filly RA, Laing FC, Mack LA, Zarutskie PW. Ectopic pregnancy. Diagnosis by sonography correlated with quantitative HCG levels. *J Ultrasound Med*. 1987;6(3):145-150.

300. Atri M, Leduc C, Gillett P, et al. Role of endovaginal sonography in the diagnosis and management of ectopic pregnancy. *Radiographics*. 1996;16(4):755-774; discussion 775.

301. Silva C, Sammel MD, Zhou L, Gracia C, Hummel AC, Barnhart K. Human chorionic gonadotropin profile for women with ectopic pregnancy. *Obstet Gynecol*. 2006;107(3):605-610.

302. Silverman NS. ACOG Practice Bulletin No. 193 Summary: Tubal Ectopic Pregnancy. *Obstet Gynecol*. 2018;131(3):613-615.

303. Barnhart K, Mennuti MT, Benjamin I, Jacobson S, Goodman D,

Coutifaris C. Prompt diagnosis of ectopic pregnancy in an emergency department setting. *Obstet Gynecol.* 1994;84(6):1010-1015.

304.   Barnhart KT, Simhan H, Kamelle SA. Diagnostic accuracy of ultrasound above and below the beta-hCG discriminatory zon *Obstet Gynecol.* 1999;94(4):583-587.

305.   Connolly A, Ryan DH, Stuebe AM, Wolfe HM. Reevaluation of discriminatory and threshold levels for serum β-hCG in early pregnancy. *Obstet Gynecol.* 2013;121(1):65-70.

Made in the USA
Middletown, DE
26 July 2019